C. Leigh B

Health and Healing
with
Bee Products

Boost health, treat conditions and prevent disease with:

- Bee Pollen
- Propolis
- Honey
- Royal Jelly

alive books

Vancouver
Canada

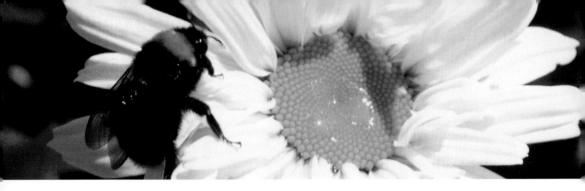

c o n t e n t s

Note: Conversions in this book (from imperial to metric) are not exact. They have been rounded to the nearest measurement for convenience. Exact measurements are given in imperial. The recipes in this book are by no means to be taken as therapeutic. They simply promote the philosophy of both the author and *alive* books in relation to whole foods, health and nutrition, while incorporating the practical advice given by the author in the first section of the book.

Recipes

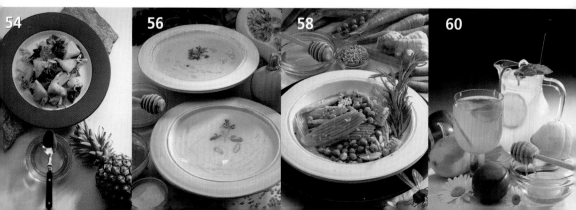

54   56   58   60

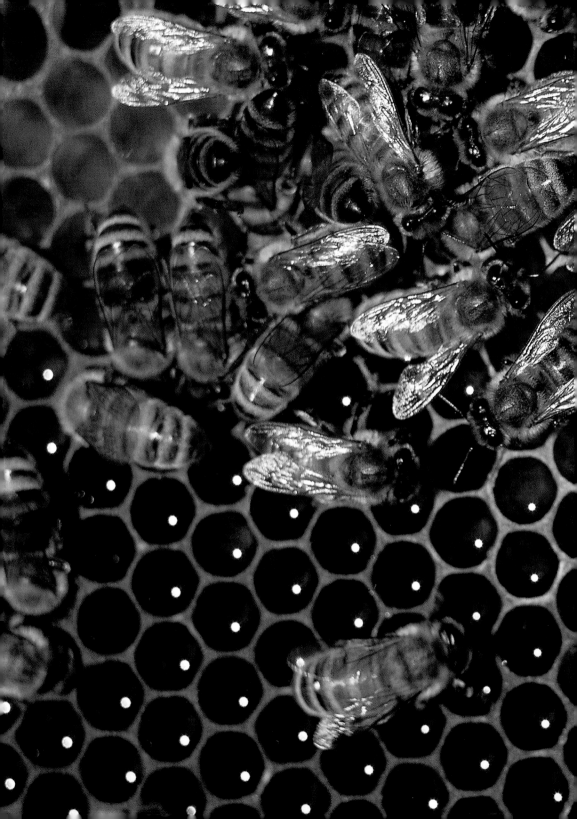

Many healing and
health-promoting
opportunities for
humans begin with
the busy honey bee.

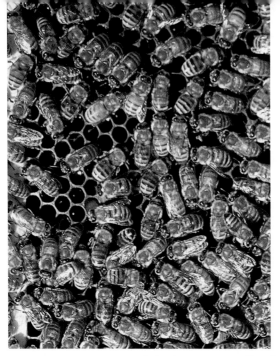

The natural healing of today's bee products comes straight from the products of the honey bee.

Introduction ....

As a child, my great uncle kept bees in his back yard on the outskirts of town. Now and then, my grandfather would take one of his brother's hives home with him.

It was there, on my grandfather's farm, that I first learned how bees live and how to care for a beehive. I learned how enjoyable chewing chunks of wax comb can be, savoring that fresh, sweet honey, straight from the source. I began to learn a little bit as well about some of the lore surrounding bee products and health–healing properties, relief from allergies, nutritional benefits.

Unfortunately, with so much other farm work to attend to, my grandfather didn't keep his bee colonies going for more than a few years.

Many years later, as a graduate student at the University of Arizona, Tucson, I was slowly beginning to realize that, even on the campus of a major research university, standard medicine really had very little to offer people like myself–young and otherwise healthy, people who really could use some help coping with the stress, late hours and fatigue, the poor eating habits, alcohol overindulgence and lingering infections that plague students.

And so I began to educate myself, and to visit some local health food stores. Then one day I listened to an absolutely compelling interview on a local radio talk show. The guest that day was Royden Brown, founder of CC Pollen Company, and he was speaking from the heart about the benefits of bee pollen.

As Mr. Brown related a story about how beekeepers in Central Europe were living to see the century mark and beyond without ever having seen a doctor, I couldn't help but recall with sadness that it was ten years since my grandfather had died, his body wasting slowly and painfully away with cancer. Meanwhile his brother, the beekeeper, was still going strong.

One of the points that made Royden Brown's interview so compelling was a discussion of how bee pollen can work as a medicine. Modern research has found that just like many popular herbal tonics, bee pollen is rich in important, health-giving phytochemicals. Some phytochemicals found in pollen can reduce inflammation and promote detoxification. Others are known to lower cholesterol, stabilize and strengthen capillaries, reduce inflammation, quench free radicals; and in addition they are antiviral, antibacterial and anticarcinogenic.

The high content of flavonoids, for example, is thought to be responsible for bee pollen's reputation for helping allergies and varicose veins. The best known and most common flavonoid in all seed plants is quercetin. Quercetin is concentrated in pollen, and is known to be an antioxidant, antihistamine, antiallergenic and antiasthmatic. It has proven valuable in fighting asthma, chronic obstructive pulmonary disease, bronchitis, sinusitis, colds, flus and allergies. Rutin, another flavonoid especially concentrated in pollen, is known to improve the condition and function of capillaries, which in turn helps to control or prevent varicose veins, venous insufficiency, hemorrhoids, hypertension and diabetic retinopathy.

I began more closely investigating not just pollen, but all the beehive products at my local health food store. With nothing to lose, I began taking generous doses of bee pollen and propolis every day. And it really helped–I was on my way in my quest to become stronger and healthier, and I polished off my PhD program ahead of most of my peers.

Thanks to the work of the honey bee, we can benefit from a wide range of health-promoting bee products.

I've now spent more than ten years keeping up with all the growing research into beehive products, lecturing on the subject and designing supplements. My entire family enjoys pollen, propolis, honey and royal jelly today. I eat two generous tablespoons of bee pollen every morning-and I'd recommend this practice to just about anyone.

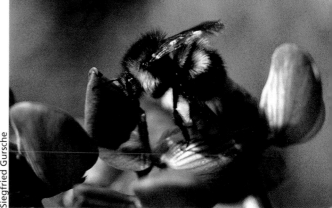

Siegfried Gursche

Bee Pollen

Bee Pollen is Super Nutritious! . . . .

To say bee pollen is nutritious is definitely an understatement. It is super nutritious! In fact, it contains nearly all the nutrients required by the human body. It is rich in enzymes and contains all the necessary amino acids the body requires.

Bee pollen contains the male reproductive material of higher plants. It is therefore a very highly concentrated source of nutrients. In fact, the nutritional composition of pollen is similar to a combination of dried legumes and nutritional yeast.

What is Bee Pollen? . . . .

Plants reproduce by pollination and plant pollen is distributed in two ways. Pollens that are dry and lightweight are dispersed through the air, carried on the winds. Other pollens are heavier because they're wetter, which makes them sticky. The sticky pollens attach themselves to visiting insects and birds, in much the same way that burrs attach themselves to a hiker's socks and pant legs.

It is the wind-borne pollens that are generally the source of pollen-induced allergies. Sticky pollens, meanwhile, are not generally associated with allergies. In fact, as we'll discuss later, the regular consumption of bee pollen can actually help provide relief from allergies for many people.

Plant pollen is a major food source for bees. It provides their protein, fat, vitamin, and trace element requirements. Worker bees travel from flower to flower, collecting pollen (of mostly the sticky variety) in special "baskets" on their legs.

Bee pollen, then, consists of a blend of plant pollen grains, collected by honeybees from a wide variety of plants. Workers

Bee pollen contains nearly all the nutrients required by the human body.

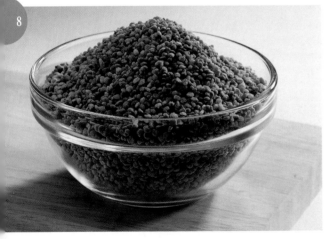

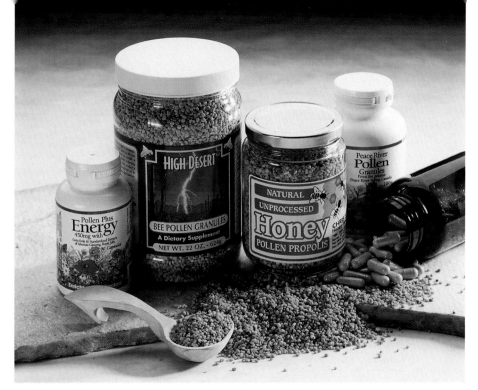

tend to collect more pollen than the colony requires. Knowing this, beekeepers have devised special screens to scrape some of the excess pollen off the bees as they enter the hive. Each of those rounded granules you may see in your jar of honey is in fact a load of pollen brushed from a bee's leg.

Among a long list of uses, bee pollen products are known to increase energy and ease allergy symptoms.

Protein

The range of protein content is quite large among various plant pollens. Bee pollen can therefore contain anywhere from 12 percent to better than 30 percent protein.

Pollen contains the complete spectrum of amino acids. Amino acids are extremely important to our health. They are the building blocks of proteins, which are needed to build every cell in the body, from blood cells to the cells in your skin, organs and bones.

Vitamins and Minerals

Vitamins and minerals are essential to life and necessary for health. Pollen contains every vitamin known to science. It is especially rich in pantothenic acid (vitamin B5), nicotinic acid (vitamin B3) and riboflavin (vitamin B2). Along with a healthy dose of B-complex vitamins, it contains vitamin C, calcium, copper, iron, magnesium, potassium and manganese. As well, more than twenty-five trace elements account for 2 to 4 percent of the dry weight of pollen. This list includes every trace element that's known to be essential for mammals.

Take note that vitamins B12 and D are quite low in bee pollen, so it should not be considered an adequate source for these vitamins (for humans, dogs or cats, or for vegan diets).

Fats

While bee pollen provides us with some essential fatty acids, we still need to supplement our diets with healthful oils such as flax, fish and hemp.

Pollen granules are 5 to 10 percent good fat by dry weight. This translates to 2 to 3 grams of fat per ounce per serving of granules (28 grams, or two rounded tablespoons). This healthful fat content contains considerable essential fatty acids, lecithin and

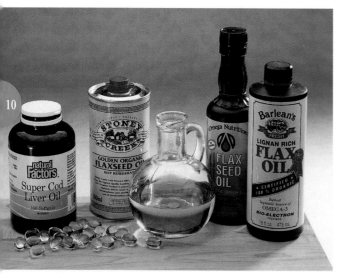

other nutrients. Essential fatty acids are essential to the body—we need them to survive because they're needed for special functions in the body aside from energy. They are also called "essential" because the body does not produce these fats themselves. Therefore we must eat them. While bee pollen gives us some essential fatty acids, we must commit to a daily supply of other healthful fats as well, such as flax oil or fish oils.

Phytochemical Nutrients

From a phytochemical (phyto = plant) standpoint, bee pollen is a powerhouse—I'd call it the ultimate "nutraceutical." Phytochemicals are a determining factor in the color and flavor of vegetables. They act as the plant's natural immune system, warding off disease and viruses. These same phytochemicals help to increase our body's immunity and help to support the body's ability to remove toxins. These protective substances have also been linked to the prevention of cancer, heart disease, diabetes and high blood pressure, to name a few.

Pollen is uniformly rich in carotenoids, flavonoids and phytosterols. The exact profile is variable, depending upon plant sources, season and growing conditions. But beta-carotene, lycopene, beta-sitosterol, quercetin, isorhamnetin, kaempferol and rutin have all been consistently reported in analyses of bee pollen.

Because pollen is typically consumed in very small quantities, the phytochemicals that are contained in it are likely to be the most important aspect of its nutritive value. These nutrients are far superior to the synthetic nutrients received from supplements. In fact, often times people who do not perceive any benefit from vitamin supplements do recognize a difference when taking bee pollen. These people may not be able to readily absorb and utilize vitamins unless they're made available in a natural food context. Clearly, we need to choose an overall nutritious diet–and bee pollen is an important component to consider including.

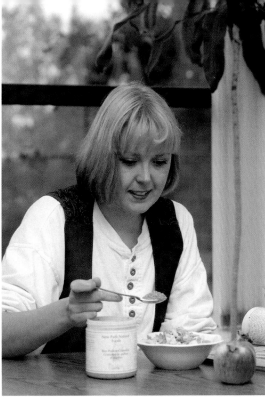

Adding bee pollen granules to a meal will increase your intake of healthful enzymes.

Enzymes

Fresh, unheated pollen also contains numerous active enzymes, coenzymes, and hormones (including growth hormones) that may be at least partially active in humans.

Enzymes are energized protein molecules, and are often referred to as the "sparks of life," because they are needed for every biological process in the body. Eating food that contains enzymes saves the body from having to make enzymes, a process that depletes energy. Eating enzyme-rich food also helps the body prevent and fight diseases such as cancer and arthritis. The antioxidant enzyme superoxide dismutase (SOD) is also commonly found in pollen.

Nutritional Impact

Chemical analyses indicate that, in theory, bee pollen is a complete and nutritious food. But does it work in practice? Try it for yourself and feel the difference. But in the meantime, we have a number of studies, such as the ones outlined below, that indicate it really does make a difference.

Added to the diets of piglets, calves, foals, adult horses, chicks, adult laying hens and pet birds, pollen has been shown to enhance growth and overall health, to increase fertility and egg production. Mice and rats have been shown to thrive on a diet of nothing but fresh bee pollen and water for periods of one month to longer than one year.

In a 1999 study out of Northeastern Ohio Universities, six female and six male rats of the same strain were fed nothing but Arizona desert bee pollen and water over the twelve-week period during which they grew to adulthood. Meanwhile, six paired male and female control rats were fed standard commercial laboratory rodent chow. The rats could eat all they wanted.

Both the males and females that were fed bee pollen remained entirely healthy. They grew and acted normally. They developed heavier brains than the controls.

But the most striking difference was that rats fed bee pollen ended up with far less body fat than rats fed lab chow. The control rats were verging on obesity at the end of twelve weeks weighing three to four times more than rats fed bee pollen.

But could it be that our featured rats weighed less because they *disliked* eating bee pollen? Not likely. Several studies have demonstrated that, given a choice between lab chow and bee pollen presented side by side, rats strongly prefer pollen. Apparently, rodents are smart enough to choose a fresh, natural whole food over processed food from a bag. So perhaps there's a lesson to be learned here for us humans!

Adding Bee Pollen to Your Diet . . . .

Bee pollen is a superior, quick and easy way to add servings of produce to your diet. One to two teaspoons of bee pollen is equivalent to a hearty serving of vegetables. So if you're always on the go, or if you don't eat all the fruits and vegetables you should, a tablespoon of bee pollen per day is a quick and easy way to dramatically improve your diet. It's a good choice for the ill or elderly, too, who perhaps can't cook, chew or digest large amounts of produce.

If you're new to trying pollen, use fresh, soft granules–and, to begin, take only a few granules at a time to make sure you're not allergic to it. Allergies to bee pollen are no more common than allergies to other foods, but they do occur. Be especially cautious if you already know you're allergic to bee stings. If you have no adverse reaction, increase your pollen intake slowly up to a tablespoonful. One to three tablespoons per day is a good range for long-term consumption.

Chewing pollen granules or tablets is the best way to eat pollen. If you can't get used to the taste, however, mix the pollen with other food, or swallow it whole with a "chaser" of something you do enjoy.

Try mixing bee pollen granules with nut butter and dry milk or hot sugar-free cocoa mix. Form the mix into balls or discs and refrigerate to harden. Or you can add bee pollen to a serving of trail mix or granola. Pollen can also be added to blender drinks and smoothies, but don't try this unless you like the taste of pollen—a little bit goes a long way!

Here are some other options, especially recommended for children, and for adults with a strong sweet tooth: Try sweetened, chewable pollen tablets and wafers; flavors include orange, honey and vanilla. A number of snack and sports nutrition bars also contain bee pollen (these typically contain less than one gram of pollen, however, whereas a tablespoon of pollen weighs 10 to 14 grams).

One to two teaspoons of bee pollen is nutritionally equivalent to a hearty serving of vegetables.

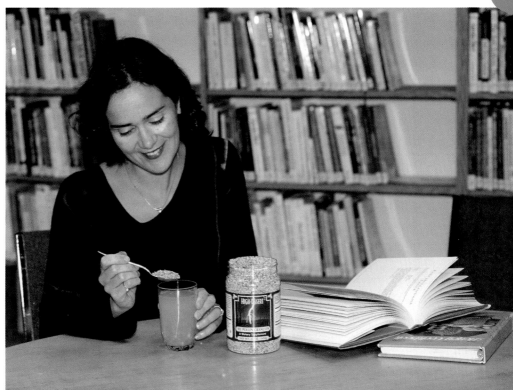

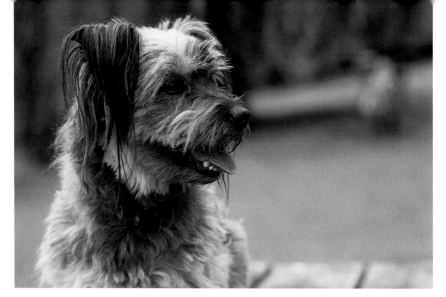

Bee pollen is not just healthful for you, but for your pet too.

Bee Pollen for Your Pets

- The majority of bee pollen consumed in North America is eaten by animals, not humans.
- Race horses are fed large amounts of pollen, particularly on days prior to big races. Compared with grazing, pollen provides high-energy nutrition, and it enables horses to conserve their energy for post time. Horses that are "off their feed," listless, easily fatigued or have poor coats tend to recover fully and rapidly when bee pollen is added to their diet.
- Bee pollen is also sold in granule, tablet or food supplement forms for dogs, cats, rabbits, ferrets and other small mammals.
- Cats are "obligate carnivores," meaning they cannot live or reproduce without animal flesh. Plant foods aren't natural components of the feline diet, so cats have a limited ability to metabolize and detoxify phytochemicals. For this reason, cats should be fed no more pollen than the manufacturer recommends.
- Dogs are more omnivorous. They can generally eat plenty of pollen, as can rodents. Too much pollen can cause loose stools in dogs, so it's wise to start with the manufacturer's recommended dose.
- Captive birds can benefit greatly from pollen supplements. Pollen likely provides dietary components that birds consume naturally in the wild, but which are lacking in commercial bird foods–or even in fresh fruits and vegetables. Adding pollen to a captive bird's diet can promote growth and enhance breeding success.

Medicinal Properties of Bee Pollen . . . .

The detoxifying and healing properties of bee pollen have been appreciated for years. Pollen has helped to alleviate allergies, fatigue, high cholesterol and triglycerides, infertility, impotence, varicose veins, recovery from illness and surgery, prostatitis and cancer.

A 1971 study done in Moscow found that 250 milligrams of bee pollen administered twice per day remarkably improved the symptoms of bleeding gastric ulcer patients. Chinese studies on humans and animals have demonstrated that consuming bee pollen or various single plant pollens several days prior to moving to high altitude reduces the incidence of altitude sickness, and apparently improves the ability to adapt to lower levels of oxygen in the air.

Yet bee pollen's use as a medicinal plant has in many ways failed to gain acceptance. Much of the older information regarding pollen has been anecdotal, uncontrolled or not referenced; however, there is ample evidence today that supports bee pollen as a valuable nutrient for the treatment and prevention of many diseases and ailments.

Bee pollen has been shown to help in a number of health and medicinal situations, including recovery from illness and surgery.

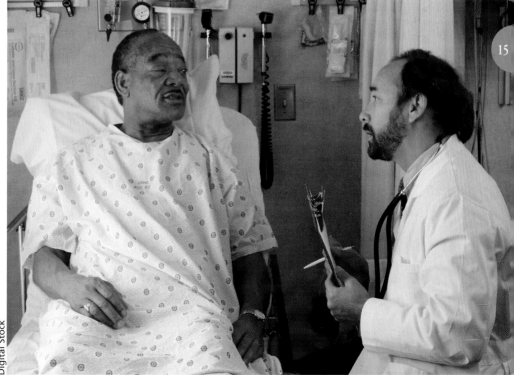

Studies Show ...

Carcinomas:

When treated with standardized pollen extracts versus untreated controls, mice with lung carcinomas survived almost twice as long. Pollen also increased the effectiveness of standard chemotherapy medications when given simultaneously.

Unlike medications, the study indicated pollen does not directly attack a tumor; instead, it stimulates the immune system.

Prostate:

The phytochemicals lycopene, beta-sitosterol, other phytosterols and numerous flavonoids contained in bee pollen have been shown to inhibit the growth of prostate tissue and to reduce pain, inflammation and the risk of prostate cancer. Also, some of the hormones in pollen may aid prostatitis as well. Studies show that standardized pollen extract is an effective treatment for prostate enlargement and prostatitis, with no significant side effects.

Liver:

Standardized pollen extracts, which are widely available in health food stores today, have been shown to protect the liver from damage and help it to detoxify.

Bee-collected pollen has also demonstrated a remarkable ability to help the process of detoxification, considerably reducing the toxic effects of aspirin, carbon tetrachloride and synthetic sex hormones in rat mothers and fetuses.

Bee pollen has proven helpful for relief from allergy symptoms, such as those caused by hay fever.

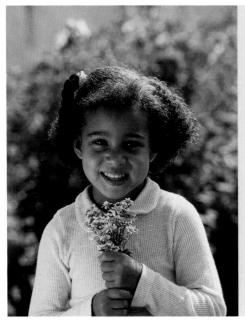

Hay Fever:

Bee pollen can help allergies. On the other hand, there's no scientific evidence to say it works like allergy shots, or that locally derived pollen is required (or even preferred). That said, there's also precious little clinical evidence available to show that *allergy shots themselves* are effective, especially considering the enormous time and expense that must be invested.

People often try bee pollen for the first time in an effort to help control pollen allergies or "hay fever." The prevailing wisdom is that consuming small amounts of bee pollen over time works like a series of allergy shots, gradually desensitizing the body to pollen exposure–the same theory that homeopathic medicine is based on. It's even been recommended to consume only bee pollen originating from your local neighborhood; presumably, you'll be eating the same pollen that's in the air around you.

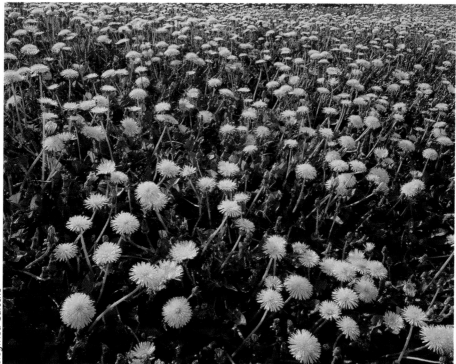

Bee Pollen and Allergies . . . .

Bee pollen is a blend of sticky pollen grains; it contains few of the wind-borne pollens that are widely allergenic (i.e., ragweed, birch, olive, various grasses).

Beekeepers select locations for their hives based primarily on access to nectar-source plants that produce tasty, clear honey. Bee-keepers also select locations near nutritious pollen-source plants that bees prefer, so that the colony remains strong.

Not all pollens are adequately nutritious for bees. In the UK, for example, some of the most nutritious pollen comes from fruit trees, dandelion, willow and clover–plants pollinated by bees. Flowering plants and bees have co-evolved, and presumably these plants found it advantageous to produce pollen that keeps bees coming back. In contrast, corn, wheat, alder, hazel and pine are wind-pollinated; they also produce pollen of inferior nutritional quality.

In general, plants that are known to produce widely aller-genic pollen do not fit the criteria used to site beehives. Quality

Some of the most nutritious pollen comes from plants pollinated by bees, such as dandelions.

Bee pollen has antiallergic, anti-inflammatory and immune system normalizing phytochemicals.

pollen manufacturers always blend pollen from different locations, seasons and/or source apiaries–so there is no single local source.

Studies have shown that high intakes of pollen (or allergy preparations containing pollen) during hay fever season help allergies more than using very small amounts throughout the year.

Meanwhile, note that the dosage of an allergy shot contains minuscule amounts of pollen antigen compared with the amount found in just one capsule of bee pollen. Bee pollen also helps alleviate allergies that are unrelated to pollen.

The large number of antiallergic, anti-inflammatory and immune system normalizing phytochemicals found in pollen are potentially responsible for the allergy benefits it produces. In this regard, bee pollen is no different than many other medicinal plants we know of that help alleviate allergies, asthma and upper respiratory infections.

Allergic to Bee Pollen?

Very few people are allergic to bee pollen, honey, propolis and/or royal jelly. These individuals need to avoid beehive products. Such allergic reactions tend to only worsen with time. A desensitizing process cannot be expected to be successful–in fact, it may be life-threatening.

These cases may entail multiple pollen allergies or they may relate to allergies to honeybee proteins. This may not be a matter of simply being allergic to bee stings; you can also be allergic to "bee dander," in the same way you can be allergic to cat, dog or cockroach dander.

Mold spores in bee products could also be the cause of allergic reactions.

Bee Pollen in History . . . .

Bee pollen in and of itself does not have a long tradition of use as a food. The widespread use of bee pollen as a food supplement can be traced back only fifty years or so, around the Second World War era.

On the other hand, of course, people have been eating bee pollen since the day they discovered honey as a food source.

Native Americans used pollen collected directly from flowers as a food source. Cattails and corn are especially prolific producers of pollen–enough can be collected to mix with flour or cornmeal to produce pollen breads and porridges. It was also used in a ceremonial manner, as a vivid yellow face paint, for example.

Honey, on the other hand, was apparently consumed in smaller amounts, as a symbolic or medicinal food.

According to the records that have survived, beekeeping was big business in ancient Egypt, Greece and Rome, throughout the Middle Ages and continuing into early-modern times in Europe. These civilizations boasted of large, professional apiaries. Landowners also tended to keep a few hives close to home to keep the household supplied.

Through the ages, beekeepers and their families probably ate more pollen than the average member of the populace, in the form of raw honey, straight from the hive. Until recently, in fact, all honey consumed came directly from the honeycomb, raw and entirely and unprocessed–and raw, unprocessed honey contains appreciable amounts of pollen. That characteristic "flowery" taste of raw honey originates directly from small amounts of plant pollen embedded in the honey.

Raw, unprocessed honey–straight from the honey comb–contains a significant amount of pollen.

Until sometime after the Industrial Revolution, sugar was a scarce commodity. Honey, however, was not. In 1996, the *British Journal of Nutrition* concluded that preindustrial Europeans ate about as much honey as they do sugar today–fifteen to thirty kilograms per year!

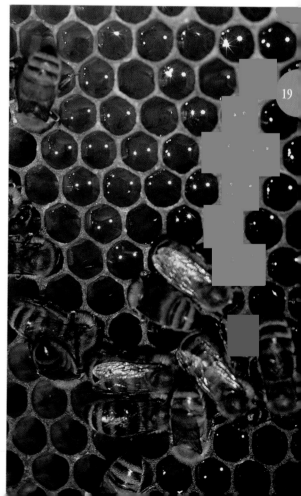

Purchasing and Storing Bee Pollen . . . .

High-quality, fresh pollen should consist of soft, pliable granules that have been neither pasteurized nor heat treated. The highest-quality bee pollen is frozen as it's collected, and stored frozen until it's packaged.

Fresh, raw pollen is in fact fresh produce, and it needs to be treated as such. Just like fresh fruits and vegetables, pollen is intrinsically variable, perishable and subject to mishandling. The granules you buy should smell and taste flowery and tart or sweet, similar to raw honey.

The best bee pollen comes from wild plant sources.

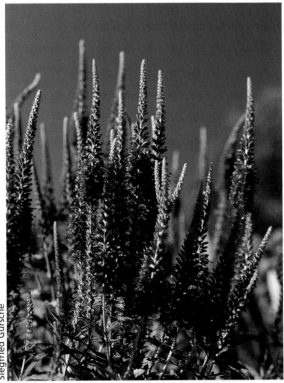

Siegfried Gursche

As mentioned previously, quality bee pollen manufacturers blend pollen from different locations, seasons and/or source apiaries. In general, the best pollen comes from wild plant sources; second best (but still excellent) originates from organic farming areas. Canadian and US manufacturers specializing in full-line bee products provide the freshest, highest-quality pollen. And Southwestern US desert plateau bee pollen has consistently proven to be the top choice (mesquite trees, among other plants, are a major source for this pollen).

Imported pollens, on the other hand, are subject to oven-drying, sterilization and longer storage durations. Oven-dried and sterilized pollens don't have active enzymes; they can also lose vitamins, polyunsaturated fatty acids and phytochemicals, and they may undergo changes in protein structure. Excessive heating or dehydration of granules makes them hard and flinty, and can render a slightly bitter taste.

Some processing of pollen is necessary because pollen grains have two tough outer coats surrounding the nutritive contents. Bees' digestive systems are designed to cope with these coats; however, the systems of humans, cats and dogs are not. Consequently, the better manufacturers gently crack pollen before it's packaged.

Granules may also, of course, be encapsulated, pressed into tablets or chewable wafers, or finely ground for use in foods and beverages. Such processing may or may not damage nutritional qualities, depending on the manufacturer.

Numerous research studies have shown that all beehive products can become contaminated with pesticides, herbicides and environmental pollutants. Fortunately, however, bees are sensitive to pollution levels. The queen bee's health apparently declines when the hive is exposed to more than it can handle; this fact limits the success of apiaries in heavily contaminated areas.

If you happen to be *mildly* allergic to bee pollen, or if you don't like the quality of a product, don't give up–send it back to the manufacturer with a letter indicating that you wish to try a different lot number. It may be that you're sensitive to just one component of the pollen blend.

Pollen should be stored in a dark, dry environment. When purchased in bulk it can be frozen for long-term storage. When sold in plastic bags, pollen should always be stored under refrigeration. Sealed containers should also be refrigerated after opening. Never add liquids or moist foods to stored pollen, and don't dip damp fingers or utensils into it.

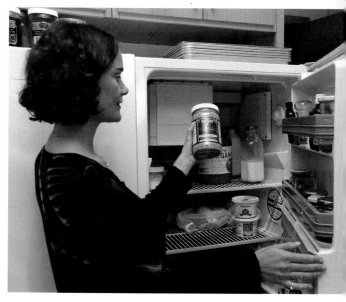

Bee pollen purchased in sealed containers and plastic bags should be stored in the refrigerator after opening.

Propolis

. . . .

For more than two thousand years, propolis has been used as an antiseptic, antimicrobial and detoxifier, treating both humans and livestock.

European, Asian and Middle Eastern cultures used propolis to heal festering wounds, bedsores, skin ulcers and jagged battle-field slashes (many weapons of war were purposefully designed to create wounds that would be difficult to suture; thus they wouldn't readily heal and became easily infected).

Anecdotal reports of the healing qualities of propolis are so numerous and convincing that researchers have formally investigated propolis to a greater extent than either bee pollen or royal jelly.

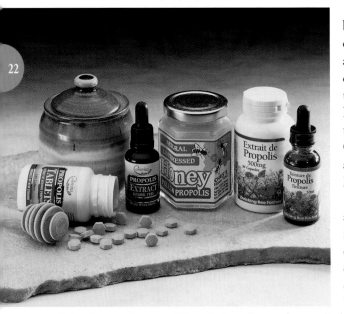

22

Most modern research has been conducted on propolis originating from temperate and northern-temperate mixed deciduous and conifer forests–the forest types found in Northern and Central Europe, the Northern US, British Columbia, Southern Ontario and Quebec and the Canadian Maritimes.

The poplar genus serves as the primary tree source in these climes. Leaf buds of poplars are known for exuding reliably large amounts of a sticky resin, often called "balsam."

Propolis has been used as an antiseptic, antimicrobial and detoxifier for more than two thousand years.

Chemical analyses of propolis have informed researchers that a chemical "fingerprint" consistently appears in the propolis of specific locales. This fingerprint is often a precise match to the resin beads collected from local trees. Bees are apparently exceedingly selective. Propolis collected in Arizona's Sonora Desert, for example, has been found to derive from a single poplar species, *Populus fremontii.*

Chemical "fingerprint" analyses also show that bees don't significantly change the resins they collect. Propolis is therefore considered an *herbal* medicine, similar to other medicinal gums and resins, such as boswellia, guggul and myrrh.

Among the hundreds of chemical compounds identified in propolis samples, researchers have found a subset of compounds that display a recurrent pattern of antiseptic, antibiotic and antifungal properties. Most of the compounds in this subset have been identified and studied in other medicinal plants as well.

Bees collect propolis from specific leaf buds and tree bark.

What is Propolis? . . . .

Propolis consists mainly of resins exuded from leaf buds and the bark of certain trees. These resins are collected by a honeybee colony's designated group of "propolis harvesters," and are then mixed with a little wax, honey and enzymes.

Bees use propolis as a kind of putty, for sealing cracks and openings in the hive and to strengthen and repair honeycombs. They also use propolis to embalm or "mummify" the carcasses of larger animals that invade the hive. Such invaders are quickly stung to death, but because the defending bees can't transport such heavy corpses away from the hive, they embalm them rather than allowing them to decay. The ancient Egyptians observed this, and used propolis as one of the embalming agents for their exquisite mummies.

It's generally believed that propolis helps to "sterilize" a bee-hive, inhibiting the spread of bacteria, viruses and fungi that would otherwise pose a significant threat in such close, humid quarters.

Antibiotic Uses of Propolis . . . .

Antibiotic drugs have been the "belles of the ball" in the post-WWII era, but the clock is rapidly approaching midnight. Overuse, and the inevitable mutations of bacteria into resistant strains, are turning antibiotics into rather dangerous "pumpkins."

Popular medical opinion and marketing campaigns advocate the use of petroleum-jelly-based ointments containing various topical antibiotics. This approach to skin wound treatment is flawed–minor flesh wounds aren't *infected*, therefore they don't *need* antibiotic treatments. And it's becoming dangerous–the constant, casual use of antibiotic ointments actually promotes the growth of antibiotic-resistant bacterial strains.

With skin bacteria that cannot be controlled, a person requiring surgery or the treatment of a larger wound is at tremendous risk for disfiguring scarring, or even life-threatening infection. The incidence of antibiotic-resistant infections in hospitals has risen dramatically–to the extent that some surgical patients must now be quarantined. We're literally returning to days gone by, when high percentages of skin wounds led to gangrene and "blood poisoning."

Fortunately, in the field of nutritional medicine, we can find some beautiful alternatives to antibiotics. The proper use of *natural* topical antiseptic products can prevent the initial growth of harmful bacteria and fungi; it has the additional benefit of actually stimulating the healing process.

So here's something you can do *right now* to help combat the rise of antibiotic-resistant bacteria: Use propolis as a topical treatment for minor cuts, sores and abrasions.

In cell culture tests, propolis extracts have been shown to significantly inhibit the growth of bacteria in the *Klebsiella pneumoniae, Escherichia coli, Staphyloccocus, Clostridium, Corynebacterium diptheriae* and some *Streptococcus* species. It is mildly active against the *Shigella, Salmonella* and other *Cornyebacterium* and *Streptococcus* species.

All of these bacteria are pathogenic, meaning that they cause common human diseases, including diphtheria, pneumonia, boils, strep throat, dysentery, scarlet fever, diarrhea, as well as wound, urinary tract, ear, sinus and throat infections. In the former Eastern Bloc countries, antibiotics have never been widely available, but beekeeping is widely practiced. To help prevent many diseases, hospitals and clinics recommend washing, gargling or irrigating the sinuses with propolis rinses, as well as taking propolis internally.

Propolis as a Wound Salve

Propolis is certainly a good weapon against bacteria when used topically. It can clearly prevent infections, and can also help heal infections that have already begun.

Propolis-Beeswax Wound Care Salve

½ heaping tsp propolis powder from capsules
6–8 soft-gel capsules vitamin A and D
4–6 400 IU soft-gel capsules vitamin E
6 1,000–1,300 mg soft-gel capsules evening primrose or borage oil
½ tsp vitamin C powder (use bulk ascorbic acid or open capsules)
⅛ tsp borax powder
2 tsp beeswax, shaved
¼ cup (60 ml) cold-pressed almond, sesame, hazelnut or olive oil
2–3 tsp glycerine or ethanol-based liquid herbal extract such as echinacea, comfrey, chamomile, yarrow and calendula, or mixed herbs (optional)
½ tsp tea tree or manuka oil (optional)

Open the propolis capsules into a small dish. Open the vitamins A, D, E and evening primrose oil capsules by carefully cutting a slit in each with the tip of a sharp knife; squeeze contents into the dish. Add the vitamin C and borax and stir until just combined; set aside.

In a heavy stainless steel or ceramic saucepan, heat beeswax and oil over low heat, swirling the pan often, until the mixture reaches 175°F (80°C). The correct temperature is reached when the beeswax liquid becomes transparent. Do not allow to boil. Remove from heat and let cool briefly until a faint haze of opaque wax forms.

Whisk the beeswax-oil mixture with a small stainless steel whisk until fully opaque with a consistency of very soft butter (about 100°F to 120°F or 40°C to 50°C). Stir in the propolis-vitamin-borax mixture. Whisk again, vigorously and continously–the mixture will initially soften but then stiffen. When the mixture is still a little soft and warm (but not hot) stir in herbal extracts and tea tree or manuka oil, if desired. Whisk until mixture is cool then pack it into several clean screw-top ointment jars and seal tightly. Refrigerate any containers you're not immediately using.

Burn Paste

This paste effectively heals burns and wounds that are infected or becoming infected. It's best to soak your wound in hot salted water, when you're changing the dressing, before applying the paste. After healing is clearly apparent (within three to seven days), use just the paste and omit soaking.

1–2 tbsp raw dark honey
1 capsule propolis
2 rounded tsp colostrum powder

Beekeepers have always treated their own wounds (and stings) on the spot with honey and propolis, and it really does work. Natural first aid for minor cuts should consist of a *natural* salve. The complex blend of compounds in propolis (and other medicinal plants) is superior to a single antibiotic in petroleum jelly.

Propolis ointments are readily available on the market. You can also purchase a tea tree or manuka oil salve, and mix in some propolis powder from opened capsules. You can even open a propolis capsule and sprinkle propolis on top of any ointment if you don't want to mix it in a salve.

Wash the wound with hot water and soap or peroxide, then blot it dry with clean tissue. Spread your ointment on the cut with clean hands or a cotton swab. Bandage it, and change the dressing regularly until the cut is well healed over (it's especially good to apply a fresh dressing before bed, because the injured area lies undisturbed and heals while you sleep).

Propolis salves are safe for children. And don't forget your pets! Note too that dogs and cats won't enjoy licking tea tree/manuka oil with propolis salve nearly as much as they seem to enjoy petroleum jelly.

Propolis as a Mouth Wash

Propolis is an effective, natural choice for many uses and ailments.

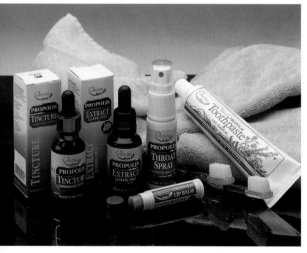

Propolis mouth rinses are astringent. They inhibit the growth of common human oral bacteria, thereby helping the body to heal oral surgery wounds and preventing halitosis (bad breath), gingivitis, tooth decay and gum disease.

A 1996 study of Israeli dental patients showed significant reductions in levels of *Streptococcus mutans* collected from their saliva after the use of propolis oral rinses. A 1994 Japanese study concluded that oral plastic surgery patients who used a propolis-alcohol rinse exhibited faster, cleaner healing, along with some reduced pain and inflammation, compared with control groups.

*Treating Upper
Respiratory Conditions with Propolis*

Propolis has been shown to be active in combating bacteria that are cultured directly from people suffering upper respiratory infections–including bacterial strains that are resistant to penicillin. Serious research began in this area because honey mixed with propolis is an ancient and apparently effective cure for upper respiratory conditions.

Antifungal and Antiviral Actions of Propolis . .

Propolis extracts are known to inhibit the growth of wood-rotting fungi. This comes as no surprise, since the trees from which propolis originates manufacture resin as a means of protecting themselves from such infection.

Brushed on the surface of cheese samples, propolis completely inhibits growth of *Aspergillus* species molds, with effects comparable to standard commercial antifungal treatments. Growth of bacteria on the cheese, including *E. coli*, was also prevented.

Accordingly, propolis inhibits growth of fungi that infect humans superficially or dermally (on the skin). The list includes *Microsporum* species, which cause ringworm and tropical skin and scalp fungal diseases, and *Trichtophyton* species, which cause common skin and nail infections.

Propolis is not considered effective against subcutaneous (below the skin or deeply embedded in the skin and nails) or systemic (internal) fungi. In cell cultures, propolis does inhibit the growth of *Candida albicans*, the culprit in common "yeast" infections, but internal use of propolis has not proven effective in alleviating chronic systemic yeast infections (in case reports, propolis has been effective when used topically for localized vaginal *Candida* infections).

Test patients with sinusitis caused by *Candida*, on the other hand, sprayed an alcohol-oil emulsion of propolis into their nostrils following a daily saline irrigation. Reportedly, nine of twelve patients fully recovered and three improved in ten to seventeen days. For persistent sinus infections, a dropper full of propolis extract added to saline water can be used for nasal/sinus irrigation.

Propolis also inhibits growth and replication of viruses in cell cultures. The list includes polio, herpes, influenza, adeno and rota viruses. An anti-herpes propolis ointment was even developed and patented, but has yet to "make it big."

Antioxidant and Detoxifier . . . .

Propolis, particularly in the form of ethanol or ethanol-water extracts, produces strong antioxidant activity–comparable to or better than well-known antioxidant herbal supplements on the market. About 50 years ago researchers noticed that bee-keepers in Central and Eastern Europe were generally healthy people, and tended to live longer than their peers. It was considered that consumption of bee products as well as the outdoor work contributed to their health and longevity.

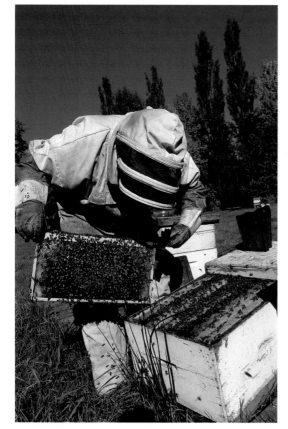

In a 1994 study conducted in Poland, identical strains of mice were given either ethanol extract of propolis daily from age thirty days on, or no propolis (the control group). The study followed two generations. Male mice receiving propolis lived longer than controls in both generations; females outlived controls in the second generation. The authors suggested that life span gains owed to the antioxidant effects of propolis extract.

About fifty years ago researchers noticed that beekeepers in Central Europe were living for 100 years or more, without ever having seen a doctor.

Other studies have positive results in relation to treatment of the liver. Detoxification of day-to-day exposure to low levels of toxins may occur when lower dosages of propolis are taken in on a daily basis. Consider it "preventing" poisoning, as opposed to treating after the fact.

Why Does Propolis Work?

- More than 180 phytochemicals found in propolis are known to have biological activity in mammals. (Biological activity refers to a substance's ability to significantly and consistently affect or alter aspects of the metabolism.)
- Flavonoids are the most abundant compounds commonly found in propolis. Flavonoids are a very large class of phytochemicals. They are ubiquitous in all seed plants, and many have documented potential health benefits.
- Clinically, propolis is considered to stimulate the growth of new tissue in addition to preventing infection. Quercetin, kaempferol, apigenin and luteolin (among other flavonoids) are known to have tissue-strengthening and regenerative effects.
- Propolis contains organic acids and their ester and alcohol derivatives. Many of the organic acids in propolis have long lists of biological activities, including anti-inflammatory, antimicrobial, antimutagenic, antihistamine, antiallergic and spasmolytic actions, and are found in numerous medicinal and aromatic culinary plants.
- Compounds identified in propolis have confirmed antifungal activities.
- Flavonoids, organic acids and their derivatives can all contribute to the antiviral effects of propolis.

Other Medicinal Uses of Propolis . . . .

Stimulating New Tissue Growth

In addition to preventing infection, propolis is believed to stimulate the growth of new tissue. Wounds heal faster and cleaner when treated with propolis salves than without. Propolis tincture has been used as a digestive aid for centuries. Case reports indicate that propolis helps heal stomach ulcers and dyspepsia, though there are no adequate controlled studies (propolis was more effective than acid blocker medications in preventing or reducing experimental stomach ulcers in animals).

Several flavonoids common in propolis are known to have tissue strengthening and regenerative effects. Propolis also contains vitamins and trace elements, which may aid in tissue healing and regeneration.

Reducing Inflammation

Propolis alcohol and water extracts and tinctures have been shown to have anti-inflammatory effects in both rodents and humans. Propolis has been reported helpful in treating arthritis, boils, acne, asthma, dermatitis, ulcers, and inflammatory bowel diseases such as Crohn's disease, irritable bowel and chronic diverticulitis. The anti-inflammatory effects increase as the dose increases, meaning that humans may need to take six to ten capsules of propolis per day to treat more severe inflammation.

Many compounds in propolis have antioxidant activity, but cell culture studies have concluded that caffeic acid phenethyl ester (CAPE) is the strongest antioxidant overall. CAPE also inhibits enzymes that play a role in exacerbating the chronic inflammation characteristic of arthritis, asthma, psoriasis and allergies.

In a 1996 British study, rats were injected with a chemical that causes acute inflammation, then treated with six milligrams per kilogram body weight of various components of propolis, reference drugs, or nothing. CAPE was the propolis component found to reduce inflammation the most, and it was nearly as effective as the reference drugs at equal doses.

Preventing Tumor Growth

The healthy beekeepers in Central and Eastern Europe also succumbed less often to cancer. Propolis phytochemicals are thought to prevent cancer development because of their antioxidant, detoxifying and antimutagenic activities. Again, the powerful CAPE has strongly inhibited the growth of skin and colon cancers in cell cultures. Propolis may help prevent cancer, and may lessen the side effects of chemotherapy and radiation treatment, but cannot be expected to effectively treat existing cancers.

How to Purchase Propolis . . . .

Variations in the content of plant resins collected around the world are quite large. Each bee colony collects propolis from its local area. For this reason, some types of bee propolis may be very beneficial, while others may be nearly worthless.

Note too that there's no standardization for propolis, as there is for other medicinal plants. Because bees are in charge of collecting the materials in propolis, humans have far less control over the outcome than we do when growing medicinal plants. But we accept this limitation, because the propolis harvester bees are doing specialized work for us, gathering and concentrating a unique herbal material that in all likelihood would be far too expensive and dangerous for humans to collect.

Most of the propolis available on the North American whole-sale market today originates in China, where the costs of producing this labor-intensive material are reasonable. Fortunately, medical research on native propolis has been carried out in China in the past, and continues today. Chinese clinical studies show that native Chinese propolis is as effective as European propolis (although more research is certainly needed).

It's important to understand that propolis research is limited to the fraction that is soluble in common laboratory solvents. The majority of the resin is *not* soluble; therefore, whole propolis products may have additional benefits or synergies that are not apparent in the soluble products.

Extracts and whole propolis capsules or tablets are both available. And both have their advantages and disadvantages. One disadvantage of commercial alcohol and water tinctures relates to the fact that they contain only the soluble fraction propolis, not whole propolis material. The advantage is that the soluble portion is more likely to be absorbed.

One disadvantage regarding whole encapsulated propolis pertains to the fact that some of the propolis simply cannot be absorbed. Even chemical compounds that are known to be absorbable may be rendered unavailable to the body if they are bound up in a gummy, insoluble resin bead.

Therefore, whole propolis that is finely ground and encapsulated may be a better choice than tablets. A newer type of propolis product is available in the form of very small propolis particles suspended in honey or syrup, designed to be taken with a spoon. This approach can combine whole ground propolis, propolis extract and other medicinal plant extracts in one palatable product. As we'll discuss in the next chapter, a raw, honey-based propolis suspension may serve as an excellent treatment for wounds, burns and skin infections.

Honey

Honey is Healing! . . . .

Honey has been revered through the ages for its healing properties. Greek, Roman, Islamic, Chinese, Egyptian, Sub-Saharan African and Native American cultures all used honey medicinally.

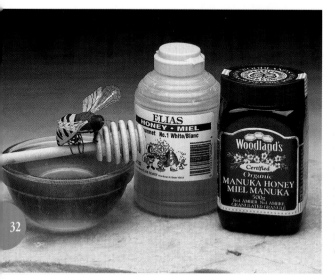

Honey has been used to treat sore throats, colds, flu, skin and stomach ulcers, diarrhea, other digestive disorders and for dressing wounds.

Recent research has confirmed the healing properties of honey. It has been demonstrated to be a broad-spectrum antibiotic, inhibiting the growth of numerous pathogenic bacteria. It's also been diagnosed as an antifungal. And antimicrobial activity is present as well, even when honey is greatly diluted. For more information on

While modern research has confirmed the healing properties of honey, it has been revered through the ages for its many uses.

honey as a food, read *Health Hazards of White Sugar* by Lynne Melcombe (*alive* Natural Health Guide #22, 2000).

A Healthful Alternative . . . .

Honey is an excellent alternative to sugar (especially white sugar) and artificial sweeteners. Bees have predigested the sugar we get in honey, which changes it to simple sugars (fructose and dextrose) and is therefore easier to digest. This naturally sweet syrup is sweeter than sugar, so not as much is needed to sweeten beverages or baked goods. It contains up to 35 percent protein and half of all the amino acids. It's also a highly concenrated source of many nutrients including enzymes, minerals and vitamins such as the B-complex, C, D and E.

Use raw honey both for consumption and medicinal use. It's extracted from the comb with a minimum of processing; it is neither overheated nor sterilized.

Raw honey contains active enzymes, vitamins and volatile chemical constituents that are destroyed or removed by heating and processing. It also contains variable percentages of bee pollen and propolis, which add vitamins and beneficial phytochemicals.

Antioxidant Activity

Floral honey can have appreciable antioxidant activity. In general, the darker a honey's color, the higher its antioxidant content will be. Water tupelo, christmasberry, sunflower and buckwheat had the highest antioxidant content in this study. But buckwheat was in a class by itself. Meanwhile, common honeys such as clover, orange, soybean and mesquite were unremarkable.

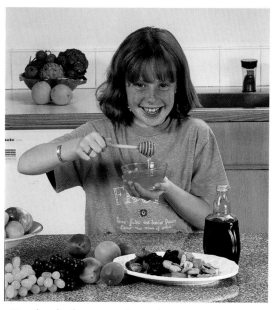

Honey is a healthy alternative to sugar and is, in fact, sweeter than sugar.

Note that you'd need to eat a lot of honey to count on it as a major dietary source of phytochemical antioxidants. In general, honey is much lower in antioxidants but much higher in sugar than fruits and vegetables. Honey, as mentioned earlier, is a healthier choice than refined sugar, but it is no replacement for tomatoes and broccoli.

Applied topically, though, honey scores highest.

What is Honey? . . . .

Honey is produced from flower nectar collected by honeybees in spring, summer and early autumn. Some bees also collect "honeydew" from the sugary secretions of aphids that feed on tree sap.

Nectar is greatly concentrated; it is stored in wax cells, thousands of which form the honeycomb. In a natural honeybee colony, honey serves as food for the bees through the winter, when plants are dormant. In an apiculture hive, most of the honeycomb is removed to extract the honey and beeswax; the

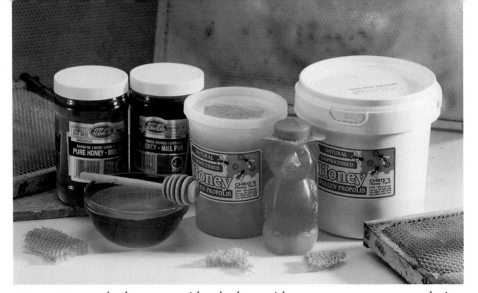

When purchasing honey be sure it is raw and unpasteurized.

beekeeper provides the bees with sugar or a corn syrup solution to sustain them.

A small percentage of honey consists of phytochemicals from the various nectar source plants. This fact creates endless variations in honey content. Unprocessed or lightly processed honey retains the flavor and aroma of its source plants. Fine honey is like fine wine–its source plants, growing location, climate zone, changes in season and weather patterns, its processing and just plain luck influence its color, aroma and flavor.

Commercial beehives, for example, may be placed in orange groves to produce fragrant, orange-scented honey, or in white clover fields to produce light, mild, all-purpose clover honey. Buckwheat flowers produce strong, dark, musky honey that's an excellent substitute for molasses in baking or barbecue sauces (be forewarned that buckwheat honey is an "acquired taste," however, if you're considering spreading it directly on your toast).

Treatment of
Skin Wounds and Infections with Honey . . . . .

Ancient warriors carried raw honey with them to treat battlefield wounds immediately. It was commonly known that cuts, abrasions or burns covered with a layer of honey would heal more rapidly, with less chance of infection. Raw honey mixed with propolis was also used.

According to a 1999 review written by Dr. Peter Molan, a noted New Zealand honey researcher, honey has been successfully used to heal thirty different types of wounds and lingering/chronic skin infections, including skin, leg, foot, varicose and diabetic ulcers; bedsores, abrasions, burns, surgical incisions, large septic wounds, cracked nipples, wounds to the abdominal wall and perineum, and gangrene.

In many cases, Dr. Molan reports, honey was "called in" to treat tough cases that weren't responding to conventional treatments. Honey was equally effective in healing large and small mammals as they recovered from veterinary surgery or experimental wounds.

The treatment of wounds with honey is associated with reductions in infection, pain, inflammation, "weeping" and foul odors. Wounds dressed with honey heal faster and more cleanly, with less scarring and better regeneration of healthy tissue. One study shows that, in more than 470 cases in which honey was used on wounds, successful healing was not achieved in just five cases (and in those five instances, the patients were extremely ill or had medical complications).

I personally mix bulk colostrum powder into High Desert raw honey with royal jelly, or raw buckwheat, manuka, or tupelo honey until I get a thick paste. Sometimes I add a capsule or two of propolis if the wound has been infected for some time. This ointment is messy of course, but it has *never* failed me, even when nothing else worked. At night, I soak wounds in hot salt water, and towel off. Then I apply the paste over the wound, dress it, and go to bed. I have treated bad burns, abscesses, pavement abrasions from bike accidents, persistent infected wounds, plastic surgeries, deep cuts, and infected insect bites with 100 percent success, and scar-free healing. Note that poorly healing wounds and/or lingering infections may require soaking and dressing two or three times per day.

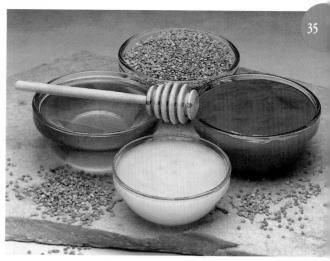

Various types of honey can be used as treatment for specific ailments and conditions.

Indeed, honey has an impressive list of clinical trials to its credit compared with most natural products. Here are some highlights:

In a 1991 clinical trial on burn patients, honey was evaluated versus a control consisting of the conventional treatment of gauze soaked in silver sulfadiazine (ss). After seven days, 91 percent of the honey-treated burns were free from infection, compared to just 7 percent for ss. After fifteen days, 87 percent of honey-treated wounds were healed, versus 10 percent in the ss group.

The study concluded that honey forms a flexible, protective barrier that prevents infection, absorbs pus and reduces pain, irritation and odors. In addition, the enzymes in honey appear to stimulate the growth of new tissue.

In two other randomized clinical trials in 1993 and 1994, honey-impregnated gauze healed burns faster than polyurethane film or amniotic membrane. Only 8 percent of forty patients treated with honey had residual scars, compared with 17 percent of twenty-four patients treated with amniotic membrane–a very expensive and specialized wound dressing compared to honey and gauze! The honey-treated burns were free from infection in seven days.

Dr. M. Subrahmanyam, the British surgeon who conducted these two studies, is a specialist in burn treatment. He has also reported the successful storage of skin grafts in honey at room temperature–a 100 percent success rate for graft uptakes after six weeks storage, and 80 percent success after twelve weeks. Treating wounds with honey prior to skin grafting operations results in better graft uptake as well.

In a 1999 study, fifty patients with wound infections following caesarean section or hysterectomy were treated with honey twice per day, or with standard antiseptic (alcohol and iodine). The twenty-six who were treated with honey were infection-free in six days, versus fifteen days for the twenty-four who were treated with alcohol and iodine. Eighty-four percent of the honey patients healed cleanly, versus 50 percent of the alcohol and iodine group. Honey treatment also reduced the average postoperative scar width by nearly two-thirds and the duration of hospitalization required by one-half. In these cases, honey actually saved the hospital and the patients money!

Treatment of Gastrointestinal Disorders with Honey ......

In a 1981 clinical trial, mixed floral honey from Saudi Arabia was the sole medication given to forty-five patients with dyspepsia (chronic indigestion). Each patient took thirty milligrams of honey prior to meals, three times daily for one month. Only eight patients reported little or no relief from dyspepsia.

Prior to treatment, thirty-seven patients had blood in their stools from bleeding ulcers–honey reduced this number to just four patients. Similarly, the number of patients with gastric or duodenal inflammation was reduced to fifteen from twenty-four, and the number of patients with duodenal ulcers dropped to two from seven.

Saudi Arabian Honey

Animal and cell culture studies have provided some clues regarding the manner in which honey protects the stomach and small intestine. In a 1997 study, floral honey from Saudi Arabia was shown to prevent increased (alcohol-induced) permeability of the blood vessels in the stomach. Increased vascular permeability is considered an initial sign of damage to the stomach lining. Blood vessels that are more permeable than normal begin to leak; eventually they break and cause gastric bleeding.

The plants known to be sources for this strain of honey include acacia, juniper, mulberry and indigo species. Previous studies on rats using Saudi honey demonstrated that it both prevented formation of stomach ulcers and healed existing ulcers (induced by alcohol and the anti-inflammatory drugs aspirin and indomethacin). It was noted as well that honey from bees fed sugar water was far less effective than natural floral honey.

New Zealand Manuka Honey

New Zealand's manuka honey is another example of a floral honey that's considered superior for medicinal use. Manuka honey has been recommended for stomach and duodenal ulcers, and case reports from physicians in New Zealand report that it is effective.

In cell cultures, manuka honey has been shown to inhibit the growth of *Helicobacter pylori*, the bacteria that often cause or contribute to the development of stomach ulcers and dyspepsia. Manuka honey is independently active against other gastrointestinal bacteria as well, including *E. coli* and *Streptococcus faecalis*.

The essential oil extracted from the manuka tree (*Leptospermum scoparium*) has also long been used topically to prevent or cure fungal and bacterial infections; to soothe diaper rash, dermatitis and psoriasis; and to kill oral bacteria when used in mouthwashes and rinses.

How to Purchase Honey . . . .

Despite its medical benefits, honey is purchased mainly for consumption as a food. Honey in general, but especially raw honey, is nutritionally superior to white, brown or "raw" cane or beet sugars, fructose and fruit sugar extracts. The sugars in honey are easily digested because the vitamins, minerals and enzymes present in raw honey aid digestion and metabolism.

The phytochemicals from the various nectar source plants create endless variations in honey content. Raw, unprocessed or lightly processed honey retains the flavor and aroma of the nectar source plants, highly variable as it may be. As noted above, raw honey is also the best choice for medicinal use. Highly processed "supermarket" honey, meanwhile, is bland and generic.

Raw and Unpasteurized

When purchasing honey ensure that it is raw and unpasteurized. Honey on the supermarket shelf has generally been heated in order to keep it liquid. The drawback, of course, is that all enzymes and some vitamins are killed by this process. Unpasteurized honey has the ability to crystalize. You might even see some pollen floating on top, which look like dirt particles, but are, in fact, very healthy. To liquefy honey, simply place the jar in a pot or bowl of hot water.

Have you ever wondered how a honey can be specific to a certain type of honey? After all, don't the bees visit many blossoms during their daily collecting trips? By law, in order for a honey to be designated *unifloral* (meaning that the honey is labeled as originating from a single floral source-clover, sunflower, orange, tupelo, etc.), just 51 percent of the nectar (or 45 percent of the

> Honey designated as *unifloral* means 51 percent is from a single floral source, such as the sunflower.

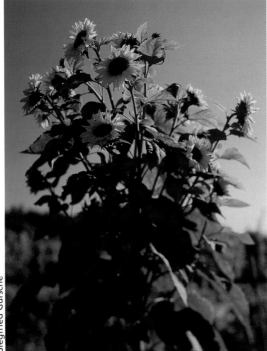

Siegfried Gursche

traces of pollen contained in the honey) must derive from the designated source plant. There's no way to control bees more closely than this!

A good way to learn more about which honeys appeal to you is to visit a farmer's market or a natural food store in an area that's known for its apiculture. Arizona, Texas and the Okanagan Valley in British Columbia are good examples, but you'll find quality beekeepers in more places than you might think. Many beekeepers earn income by renting their bee colonies to farmers and orchardists when certain crops and trees are flowering. The hives are transported to locales where crops are in bloom and the bees are willing to "work for food"–gathering nectar and pollen while also pollinating the local crops.

So you may find some "samplers" to taste at your local farmer's market or natural food store. These places are also a good resource for consulting with knowledgeable people willing to help you choose a honey that will appeal to you and your family.

After opening, a container of honey can be stored sealed, out of direct heat and light at room temperature, for at least four to six months. A kitchen cabinet is a good storage location. If you buy honey in bulk, or if your weather/climate is quite warm, you might want to keep a small jar on the shelf and refrigerate the remainder until needed.

If you have a problem with ants in your home, you may need to store honey in the refrigerator. You can also try keeping the entire jar sealed inside a tin or plastic container with a tight-fitting lid.

"Eat honey my son, it's good for your health."
–Proverb 24.13

Precautions Regarding Honey

Because approximately 80 percent of honey consists of glucose and fructose, honey is a concentrated source of simple sugars. Excessive consumption is not recommended for anyone who has diabetes, abnormal glucose tolerance, hypertension or obesity.

Although raw and unpasteurized honey is relatively sterile, some hardy bacterial and fungal spores can occur (unpasteurized honey cannot be heated as that would destroy the natural complex of the honey, and it would no be considered a whole food).

Minor amounts of spores in honey pose no risk for adults, or even toddlers. But small infants may suffer serious infections–botulism, in particular. Botulism spores don't germinate inside adult humans or children, because our stomach acid kills them. Infants, on the other hand, don't produce strong stomach acids, thus spores can germinate in their intestines. Therefore children less than one year should never be fed honey of any kind.

Approximately 95 percent of all reported infantile botulism cases occur in infants under thirty-five weeks of age. And far more cases are traced to breast milk and corn syrup than they are to honey ingestion (similarly, unpasteurized juices, corn syrup and low acid home-canned foods should never be fed to infants).

Honey used topically to treat minor wounds and infections poses little botulism risk, unless it can be licked off. Bandage wounds tightly, and don't apply honey to a baby's fingers or toes.

Royal Jelly

Royal Jelly Prevents Disease . . . .

Taking a cue from the queen, traditional Chinese medicine recommends consumption of royal jelly, describing it as "food of the emperors." Considered mysterious and exotic, royal jelly has traditionally been believed to prolong life, prevent disease and return the vitality of youth to the aged. It is especially prized by Asian cultures.

Use Royal Jelly for ...	
• Anorexia	• Hair loss
• Anxiety	• Impotence
• Arteriosclerosis	• Liver disease
• Arthritis	• Pancreatitis
• Bone fractures	• Insomnia
• Bronchial asthma	• Kidney disease
• Depression	• Seborrhea
• Dermatitis	• Stomach ulcers
• Eczema	• Varicose veins
• Fatigue	• Skin disorders
• Lack of sexual desire in women	• Weakened immune system

Many health claims have been made regarding royal jelly; they range from curing everything from acne to infertility. But almost all of this information is anecdotal. Outside of Asia, very little medical research has been done on royal jelly.

This fact doesn't necessarily imply that fresh, high quality royal jelly is ineffective; it simply recognizes the fact that there really hasn't been much incentive for investigation. In China, royal jelly is financially competitive with pharmaceutical medicines, so more clinical research happens there. In China, Russia and former Eastern Bloc countries, royal jelly has been successful in treating stomach ulcers, varicose veins, impaired circulation, impotence, dyspepsia, loss of normal sexual interest, fatigue, anorexia and chronic viral and bacterial infections.

In general, however, royal jelly's reputation for returning vitality to the aged can be substantiated at least to some degree by research, which has demonstrated that this substance does help prevent disease.

Why Does Royal Jelly Work Medicinally?

A big part of staying "young at any age" means maintaining healthy cardiovascular and immune systems. A unique fatty acid in royal jelly called HDA may act to inhibit blockage and hardening of the arteries, and blood clot damage to the artery walls. Royal jelly contains all the B vitamins as well as phytosterols, acetylcholine and hormones, all of which work together to lower cholesterol and help prevent heart disease. And HDA, antimicrobial proteins, enzymes and gamma globulin all play a role in royal jelly's ability to prevent infection and stimulate normal immune responses.

Royal jelly constituents known to help heal wounds, dyspepsia and stomach and duodenal ulcers include pantothenic acid, phytosterols, certain flavonoids, fatty acids and, in some cases, enzymes.

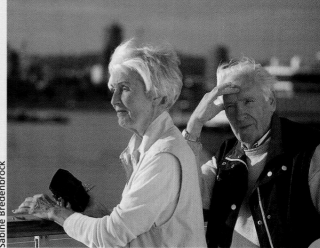

Sabine Bredenbrock

Royal jelly helps people stay young by maintaining healthy cardiovascular and immune systems.

What is Royal Jelly? . . . .

Royal jelly is the primary food bees produce to develop larvae in the beehive. Unlike other hive products, royal jelly is not a plant product, collected and modified by bees; it is a substance that bees actually manufacture. Nurse bees ingest pollen and nectar. They then secrete royal jelly from special glands in their heads–sort of a honeybee "milk."

All larvae are fed royal jelly for three days. The overwhelming majority, those destined to become worker bees, are then cut off. Only the queen larvae continue to be fed royal jelly throughout her life. It is this rich diet of nothing but royal jelly that transforms the queen into a sexually mature powerhouse, living five to seven years and laying more than her weight in eggs daily. By contrast, worker bees are sterile, their lives span only seven to eight weeks and they remain 40 to 60 percent smaller and lighter than their queen.

Royal jelly is not produced in abundance like honey. It is also expensive and labor intensive for beekeepers to harvest. With

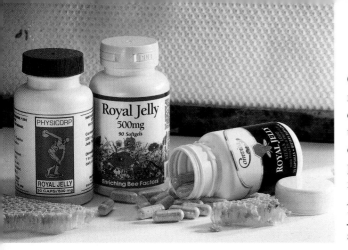

China's inexpensive labor market, that country makes extensive use of natural products for primary health care; consequently, royal jelly production is a bigger business there than it is in North America. Korea, Taiwan, Japan and Australia also have sizable royal jelly industries.

Royal jelly has traditionally been used to prolong life, prevent disease and recapture the vitality of youth. It has many modern uses.

The Composition of Royal Jelly . . . .

Fresh royal jelly is roughly 66 percent water, 15 percent carbohydrates, 13 percent protein, 5 percent fat, and 1 percent trace elements.

Royal jelly's carbohydrates are mostly fructose and glucose. The complete spectrum of amino acids exist in the protein and free amino acid fractions. The fat fraction contains a mix of polyunsaturated, monounsaturated and saturated fatty acids, including linoleic and alpha-linolenic acids, acetylcholine, lecithin and related phospholipids.

Royal jelly contains all the B vitamins, and it is particularly rich in pantothenic acid. It contains traces of vitamins A, C, D, E and K. While royal jelly is a balanced, nutritious food, it's not normally consumed in quantities greater than a gram or two per day. Royal jelly is sometimes recommended as a complete amino acid supplement for vegans, or as a source of essential fatty acids. This fact can be misleading, however, because the quantities of royal jelly ingested are so minute that the basic protein, carbohydrate and fat content is in fact inconsequential.

In the majority of cases, then, we must turn to the minor components of royal jelly in order to account for any health benefits. It is these minor components, combined with the rich nutrient mix, which turn an ordinary larva into a queen, greatly prolonging her life.

Immune System Factors

One of the functions of milk produced by humans and other mammals is to help in initiating normal immune responses in newborns. It's believed that royal jelly serves a similar function for bee larvae. Unique proteins secreted by the nurse bees into the royal jelly are believed to play an important role in defending against infectious agents and toxins. At low concentrations (comparable to pharmaceutical antibiotics) the protein royalisin, has been found to be highly effective against cultures of bacteria that infect bees, humans and other mammals. Apisin, a royal jelly protein linked to a sugar, has been observed to stimulate the growth of human immune cells in culture.

We do need to bear in mind that the overwhelming majority of honeybees don't outlive two months. The immune protection that bee larvae require as *individuals*, therefore, is rudimentary compared with the needs of a human infant. But protection of the bee *colony as whole* is a different matter. Infections or toxins that prevent normal development of larvae will ravage the colony.

The queen, in particular, must be protected from infection and premature aging–or the colony will perish. Should the need arise for a new queen, nurse bees are always tending to larvae, ready to replace her. The queen's lifetime diet of royal jelly is the best example of an immune-boosting, anti-aging "power food" that I can think of! Keep in mind it is the royal jelly *alone* that makes the queen. It may be concluded, then, that royal jelly consumption–whether it's for three days or a lifetime–evidently plays some role in the colony's "collective immunity."

Antibiotic and Antiviral Factors
Royal jelly collected from larvae three days old has been found to be the highest quality and exhibits the greatest antimicrobial activity (coincidentally or not, it's also produced in greatest abundance on the third day). In a 1995 Egyptian study, a suspension of three-day royal jelly in water completely killed cultures of *Staphylococcus aureus*, and killed 71 and 83 percent respectively, of *Bacillus subtilis* and *E. coli* cultures in three hours. The effect was augmented by mixing honey with royal jelly–*S. aureus* could not be detected in the culture plate after just two hours of exposure to honey plus royal jelly.

In the midst of an influenza epidemic in Sarajevo, Yugoslavia, just 9 percent of a group of hospital patients who took daily doses of royal jelly developed flu, compared with almost 40 percent of untreated patients (unfortunately, the dosage was not specified). Prevention of influenza may be at least partially due to an immune-stimulating effect of royal jelly.

Lowering Cholesterol

A 1995 review of controlled human and animal studies concluded that, in humans, 50 to 100 milligrams of royal jelly (dry weight) per day decreased total serum cholesterol by 14 percent, and lipids by 10 percent. Most humans in the studies reviewed received royal jelly by injection, but injected doses were found to be only slightly more effective than oral doses. Royal jelly supplementation also slowed the development of blockage and hardening of the arteries in rabbits fed very high-fat diets.

Royal Jelly for the Skin . . . .

For centuries, royal jelly has been applied to soften skin, remove wrinkles and heal eczema and dermatitis. Its natural ingredients can blend with and fortify the skin's natural hydroxy fatty acids. It's not commonly appreciated that polyunsaturated fatty acids are mainly converted to hydroxy fatty acids by the skin cells. The exact purpose of these natural hydroxy fatty acids is to protect the skin from dehydration, irritation, and inflammation. Hydroxy fatty acids take up water and bond with it, thereby "holding" water in the skin and preventing it from evaporating.

Royal jelly has softened skin for centuries.

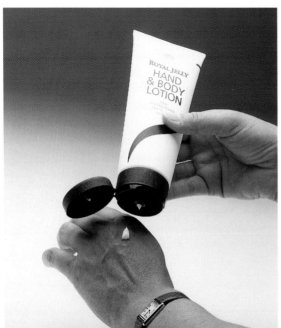

The elements contained in royal jelly can be directly absorbed and utilized by the skin. All of these qualities indicate that *concentrated* royal jelly can be an effective treatment for moisturizing the skin and soothing dermatitis. Skin products with traces of royal jelly, however, cannot be expected to provide much benefit. Ancient Egyptian queens rubbed pure royal jelly into their skin—a real luxury. Personally,

44

I have used fresh undiluted royal jelly or freeze-dried royal jelly mixed with evening primrose oil and vitamin E under eyes, on dry skin patches, and on healing cuts to minimize scarring.

Royal jelly has an immune-stimulating effect.

I recommend royal jelly (fresh or dried) mixed with evening primrose and calendula extract for treating itchy, scaly eczema and dermatitis. Other appropriate soothing herbal extracts or essential oils (such as licorice, lavender, propolis, yarrow and chamomile) can be added as desired, but don't dilute the royal jelly too much. You may want to use an anti-inflammatory herbal wash during the day, and rub in a royal jelly/oil mixture at night. Proportions do not need to be exact. For example, mix together 2 tablespoons of fresh royal jelly, 2 teaspoons liquid herbal extract and 2 teaspoons evening primrose or borage oil (apx. ten 1000 mg capsules of oil squeezed out). Add a total ¼ teaspoon of essential oil(s) if desired. Mix into a thick liquid; adjust proportions as needed to get desired consistency, but don't add more essential oils. If you are making it in bulk, cover tightly in a small jar and refrigerate, taking out to use as needed. A week's worth can sit on the shelf to be used daily if you don't like it cold.

How to Purchase and Use Royal Jelly . . . .
Royal jelly is synergistic with other bee products. It can be effective, for example, when taken in combination with propolis and honey for alleviating ulcers and viral infections. It may be useful, taken along with bee pollen, as a highly absorbable natural vitamin supplement.

Be sure to sample a tiny amount of royal jelly the first time you try it. There is no risk known for doses between 2 and 20 grams per day. One to two grams of liquid royal jelly is a good daily preventive dose. One gram of liquid royal jelly is roughly equivalent to 200 to 300 mg freeze-dried (the amount typically packaged in one capsule or tablet). You can double or triple this dosage if you're elderly, immune-suppressed, or if you're recovering from illness or injury. There have been reports of royal jelly causing breathing difficulties or asthma attacks in sensitive persons. It's possible you may be allergic to specific bee proteins in royal jelly, even if you don't react to honey, bee pollen, propolis or bee stings.

Pure royal jelly is quite perishable, and cannot be heated or exposed to light. The highest quality products come from manufacturers who offer a full line of bee products.

Fresh royal jelly can be purchased as a liquid or as soft-gel capsules stored under refrigeration (there should be an expiration date on the bottle). Don't purchase vials of royal jelly that have been stored at room temperature for an indeterminate period. Poorly marked, undated vials are often imported from Asian countries; and if no manufacturer is listed, you'll have no direct contact information in case you have questions or aren't satisfied with the product.

Royal jelly can be successfully freeze dried, which keeps it fresh, viable... and stable at room temperature.

Fresh royal jelly is also often sold mixed with honey. Honey is a natural preservative for this product; it will protect it quite well if the honey is stored tightly capped and out of direct heat and light. After opening, honey with royal jelly can be stored at room temperature for several months. If you don't use it up quickly, however, or if the weather/climate is hot, it's best to refrigerate it after opening.

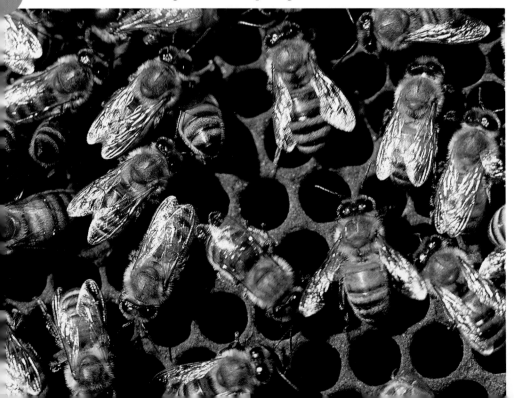

Respect the Honey Bee

I have the deepest respect and affection for this most incredible of creatures–the honeybee (*Apis mellifera*). I have been involved in apicultural, apitherapeutical and apipharmaceutical research now for more than a quarter of a century. The more I learn about the bee itself, its society and about bee products, the more I admire this wonderful creature.

At the same time, I realize how indebted we are to bees, and to which extent their products are underused, understated and misunderstood. It's time to get serious about these treasures from the beehive. Above all, however, it is time to show more respect and appreciation for those tireless creatures who provide these materials to us.

> "Unique among all God's creatures, only the honeybee improves the environment and preys not on any other species."
> –Royden Brown

Every time I open a beehive in our research apiary, I can't help but pause and quietly admire these wonderful little beings who are purposefully fulfilling their role in the grand scheme of things. It is so unfortunate that after all the honey bee has provided man, we are not reciprocating this goodness or offering much protection in return.

All the subspecies of *Apis mellifera* worldwide are in danger today. In fact, both amateur and professional beekeeping is collapsing on a global scale, which is very sad, and bad news for humanity since we so greatly depend on the pollination of the honey bee. The dangers to the honey bee are man-made and are literally threatening the very existence of this lovely, peaceful and important creature.

The threats include pesticides and insecticides, introduction of Asian Varroa mite to honey bee colonies, "importation" of new and exotic diseases to our bee, introduction and spread of extremely aggressive AHB (Africanized honey bees to the Americas) and more.

As a member of the research team for Natural Factors, I am delighted to report that we are very much interested in and committed to the well-being of the honey bee.

It is not just apipharmacological research and utilization of bee products by Natural Factors, but above all it is the commitment to apicultural research, investing in the well-being of the source of these unique products. Please respect the honey bee.

by Jan V. Slama MSc.
Research Scientist
Natural Factors Nutritional Products Ltd.

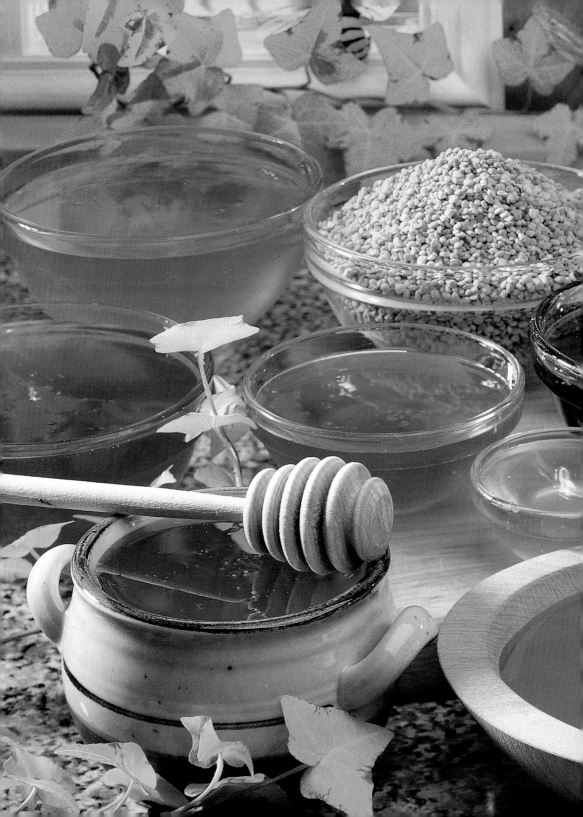

Let the honey bee's
magic into your kitchen
for both taste and health.

Honey-Pollen-Fruit Smoothies

Your kids will enjoy these rich and tasty smoothies and won't have a clue that they're drinking all the essential amino acids, minerals, vitamins and fats they need to grow strong and healthy.

2 cups (500 ml) **organic whole milk**

2 cups (500 ml) **peaches, raspberries, kiwi or fruit of your choice, chopped**

1 tbsp unpasteurized honey

1 tbsp bee pollen granules

1 tsp freshly squeezed lemon juice

Fresh mint, for garnish

Place all ingredients in a blender and blend until smooth. Garnish with mint and serve.

Serves 2

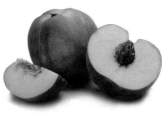

peach

Pear-Cardamom Smoothie

2 cups (500 ml) **organic whole milk**

2 cups (500 ml) **pear, peeled and chopped**

1 tbsp unpasteurized honey

1 tbsp bee pollen granules

1 tsp freshly squeezed lemon juice

Pinch cardamom, ground

Fresh mint, for garnish

Place all ingredients in a blender and blend until smooth. Garnish with mint and serve.

Serves 2

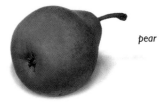

pear

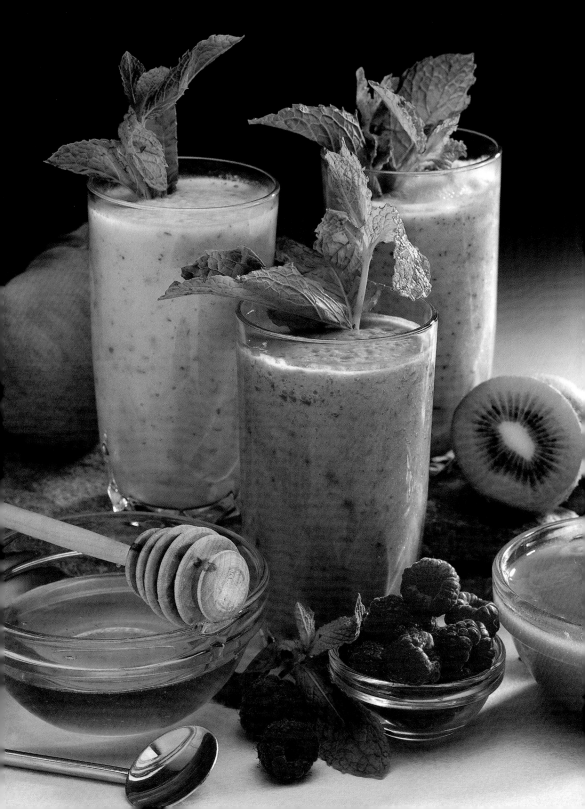

Millet Puff Bars with Bee Pollen

Cut this delectable and healthy cereal treat into small squares, pour milk over top and serve it for breakfast. It also makes a wonderful snack or a tasty dessert. Millet puffs are available in health food stores. Don't be afraid to adjust amounts as you go along or add different ingredients, such as dried fruit. You may need to add a little more honey if the results are too dry, or a bit more cereal if too wet.

2 cups (500 ml) **millet puffs**

2 tbsp hazelnuts, freshly ground

2 tbsp bee pollen granules

1 tbsp flax seeds

½ cup (125 ml) **unpasteurized honey**

2 tbsp butter

½ tsp vanilla or almond extract

2 tbsp sesame seeds

In a bowl, combine millet puffs, hazelnut, bee pollen and flax seeds; set aside.

In a pot, combine honey and butter and heat until it starts to bubble. Remove from heat and stir in vanilla extract. Pour over millet puff mixture and mix thoroughly with a wooden spoon.

Place mixture in a 9"x 9" (23 cm x 23 cm) pan and, using wet hands, press the surface until mixture is even. Sprinkle sesame seeds over top and press again. Let cool until solid.

Cut in squares and serve.

Makes 16 squares

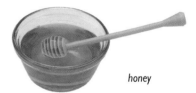

honey

> ### Pollen Preference
> Start with a smaller amount of bee pollen if you or your kids are just getting used to it–you can always press more bee pollen into the tops of the bars later.

> ### Dried Fruit Option
> If you want to make a fruit bar with dried fruit, use orange extract instead of the vanilla extract.

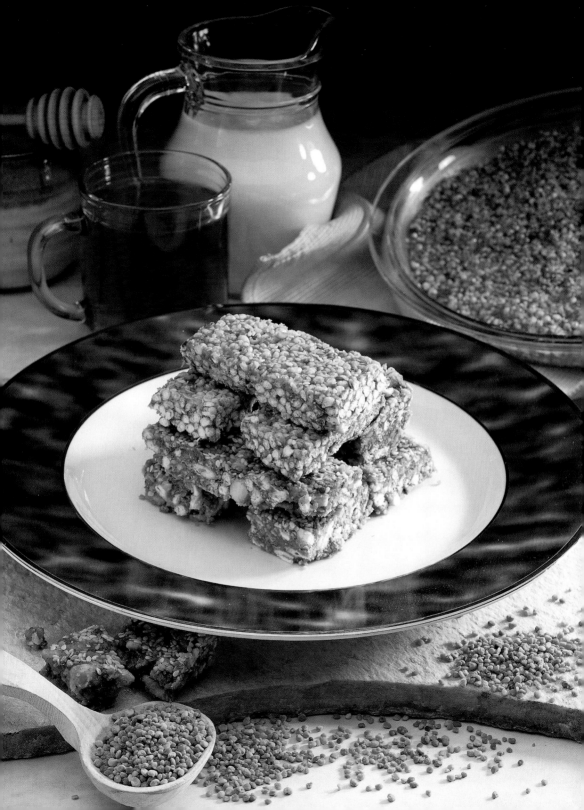

Warm Pineapple-Baby Bok Choy Salad

What does "Let's meet in the middle" mean? This dish is a negotiation between the unique texture and flavor of the baby bok choy and the sweet and sour taste of pineapple–a wonderful taste combination full of vitamins and minerals.

1 lb (500 g) **baby bok choy**

1 cup (250 ml) **fresh pineapple, cut in chunks**

2 tbsp butter

2 tbsp green onion, chopped

1 tbsp unpasteurized honey

Pinch ground cinnamon

1 tsp black and white sesame seeds

Blanch the baby bok choy in a pot of salted boiling water for 3 to 5 minutes. Drain and rinse in cold water. Chop bok choy into pieces then sauté in butter. Add pineapple, green onion, honey and cinnamon and sauté for 3 more minutes.

Garnish with sesame seeds and serve.

Serves 2

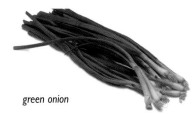

green onion

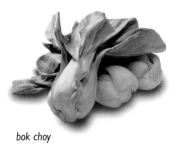

bok choy

Ripe Test
Pick up the pineapple by one of its green leaves. A leaf that comes off easily is a good sign that the pineapple is ripe. Don't heat the pineapple too long, otherwise its valuable enzymes will be destroyed.

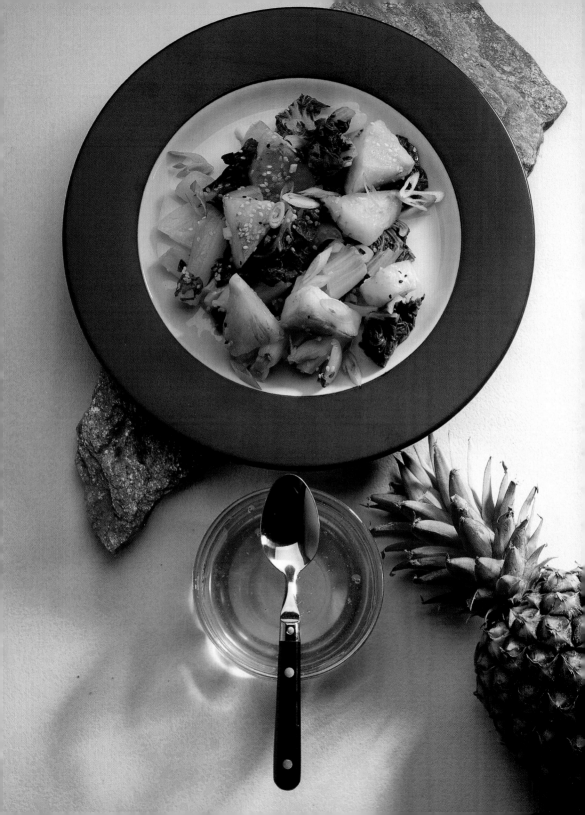

Pumpkin-Honey Soup

After a tiring day's work, this soup's unforgettable combination and taste will comfort both your body and soul. The lemon juice gives extra zest; make sure you add it at the end so the heat doesn't destroy the vitamin C.

2 cups (500 ml) **pumpkin, cut in 1"** (3 cm) **cubes**

1 medium sweet potato, peeled and cut in 1" (3 cm) **cubes**

½ cup (125 ml) **carrot, cut in 1"** (3 cm) **cubes**

½ white onion, diced

2 tbsp extra-virgin olive oil

3 cups (750 ml) **vegetable stock or water**

1 tbsp + ½ tbsp unpasteurized honey

Pinch white pepper

Pinch sea salt

2 tbsp butter

1 cup (250 ml) **kefir or buttermilk**

1 tsp fresh lemon juice

Fresh cilantro, chopped, for garnish

Heat oil in a large pot and sauté pumpkin, sweet potato, carrot and onion for 3 to 4 minutes until tender. Add vegetable stock, 1 tablespoon of honey and seasonings; cook for 15 minutes until all ingredients are soft. Place soup in a blender and slowly add kefir while blending. Blend until smooth and velvety. Return to pot, stir in butter and lemon juice and keep warm.

Pour soup into bowls, drizzle with remaining honey, sprinkle with cilantro and serve.

Serves 4

pumpkin

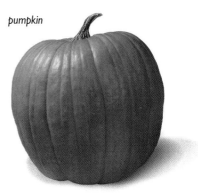

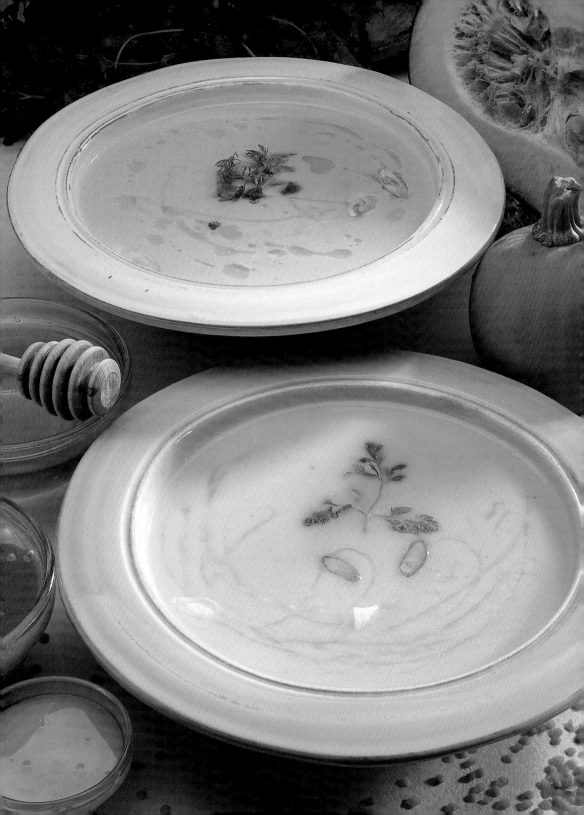

Honey-Glazed Vegetables

Eating carrots and peas together is usually a bore, however with this recipe you'll want to have them all the time. The carrots, a source of vitamins A and E, along with the vitamin C in the orange juice, will fully satisfy your body's need for antioxidant vitamins.

2 cups (500 ml) **carrots, sliced**

1 cup (250 ml) **vegetable stock or water**

1 cup (250 ml) **fresh peas**

¼ cup (60 ml) **orange rind**

½ cup (125 ml) **orange juice**

3 tbsp unpasteurized honey

2 tbsp butter

Fresh rosemary, for garnish

Cook carrots in vegetable stock for 5 minutes or until liquid is reduced by two-thirds. Add peas and cook for 3 minutes. Add orange rind and juice, honey and butter; cook for 3 to 5 minutes longer.

Place vegetables on plates, garnish with rosemary and serve. This dish is delightful on its own or served with rice or roasted potatoes.

Serves 2

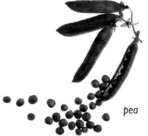

pea

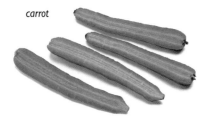

carrot

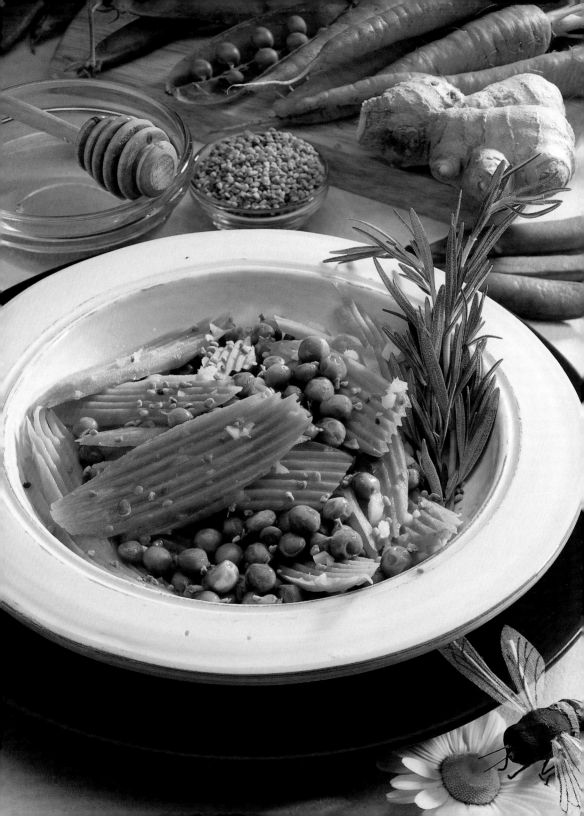

Honey Lemonade

Nothing satisfies your thirst more than this simple, humble lemonade, which can be extremely healing if you use fresh and healthful ingredients. This version nourishes the body with enzymes and vitamins B-complex, C, D and E. I use lime because it complements the honey, has a nice aroma and flavor, and is less acidic than lemon.

2 tbsp unpasteurized honey

1 cup (250 ml) **warm water**

3–4 cups (0.75–1 l) **cold water**

1 cup (250 ml) **fresh lime or lemon juice**
(about 4 large limes)

5 leaves fresh lemon balm

5 leaves fresh mint

Lime slices and rind, for garnish

Combine honey and warm water in a serving pitcher and mix until honey dissolves. Stir in cold water and lime or lemon juice then add lemon balm and mint; mix well. Garnish with lime and serve chilled over ice.

Makes about 6 cups (1.5 l)

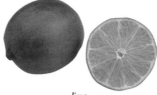

lime

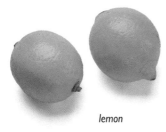

lemon

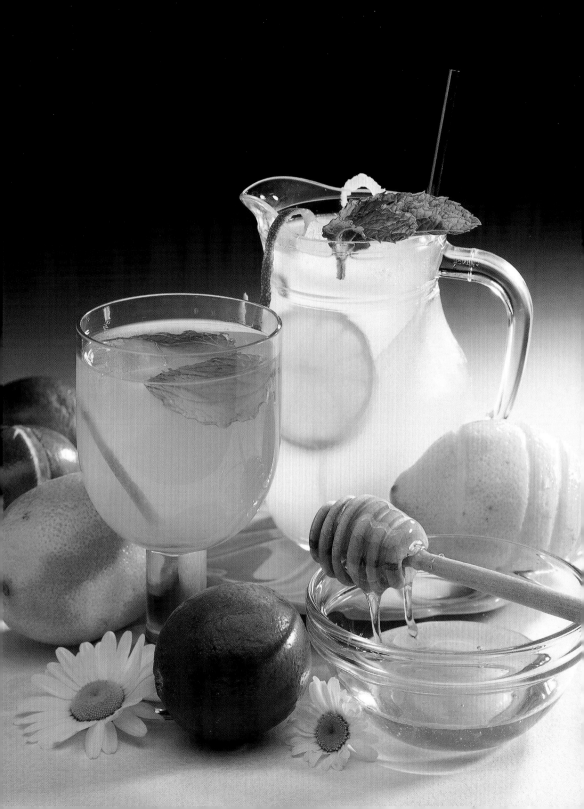

references

Bee Pollen

Bonvehi, J.S. and Jorda, R.E. "Nutrient composition and microbiological quality of honeybee-collected pollen in Spain." *Journal of Agricultural and Food Chemistry.* Vol. 45 (1997): 725–732.

——— *How to Live the Millennium: The Bee Pollen* Bible. Prescott AZ: Hohm Press, 1989.

Buck, A.C. et al. "Treatment of outflow tract obstruction due to benign prostatic hyperplasia with the pollen extract Cernilton: a double-blind placebo controlled study. *British Journal of Urology.* Vol. 66 (1990): 398–404.

Campos, M. et al. "An approach to characterization of bee pollens via their flavonoid/phenolic profiles." *Phytochemical Analysis.* Vol. 8 (1997): 181–185.

Ceglecka, M et al. "Effect of pollen extracts on prolonged poisoning of rats with organic solvents." *Phytotherapy Research.* Vol. 5 (1991): 245–249.

Furusawa, E. et al. "Antitumor potential of pollen extract on Lewis lung carcinoma implanted intraperitoneally in syngenic mice." *Phytotherapy Research.* Vol. 9 (1995): 255–259.

Juzwiak, S. et al. "Pollen extracts reduce the hepatotoxicity of paracetamol in mice." *Phytotherapy Research.* Vol. 6 (1992): 141–145.

Liebelt, R.A. "Bee pollen, a wonderful food—and a whole lot more." *American Bee Journal.* September (1994): 611–614.

Liebelt, R.A. and Calcagnetti, D. (1999). "Effects of a bee pollen diet on the growth of the laboratory rat." *American Bee Journal.* May (1999): 390–395.

Linskens H.F. and Jorde, W. "Pollen as food and medicine—a review." *Economic Botany.* Vol. 51 (1997): 78–87.

Songkun, S. et al. "Study of the anti-aging factor (SOD) in pollen." *Apiculture of China.* Vol. 50 (1997): 7–9.

Propolis

Amoros, M. et al. "Comparison of the anti-herpes simplex virus activities of propolis and 3-methyl-but-2-enyl caffeate." *Journal of Natural Products.* Vol. 57 (1994): 644–647.

Cheng P.C. and Wong, G. "Honey bee propolis: prospects in medicine." *Bee World.* Vol. 77 (1996): 8–14.

Chinthalapally, V.R. et al. "Inhibitory effect of caffeic acid esters on azoxymethane-induced biochemical changes and aberrant crypt foci formation in rat colon." *Cancer Research.* Vol. 53 (1993): 4182–4188.

Dobrowolski, J.W. et al. "Antibacterial, antifungal, antiamoebic, antiinflammatory and antipyretic studies on propolis bee products." *Journal of Ethnopharmacology.* Vol. 35 (1991): 77–82.

El-Ghazaly, M.A. and Khayyal, M.T. "The use of aqueous propolis extract against radiation-induced damage." *Drugs Under Experimental and Clinical Research.* Vol. 21 (1995): 229–236.

Focht, J. et al. "Bactericidal effect of propolis in vitro against agents causing upper respiratory tract infections." *Arzneimittel-Forschung.* Vol. 43 (1993): 921–923.

——— "The composition and plant origins

of propolis: a report of work at Oxford." *Bee World.* Vol. 71 (1990): 107–118.

Khayyal, M.T. et al. "Mechanisms involved in the anti-inflammatory effect of propolis extract." *Drugs Under Experimental and Clinical Research.* Vol. 19 (1993): 197–203.

Kimoto, T. and Kurimoto, M. "Antioxidant effects and prevention of carcinogenesis by oral administration of Brazilian propolis and Atrepillin C." *Honeybee Science.* Vol. 20 (1999): 67–74.

Magro-Filho, O. and de Carvalho, A.C. "Topical effect of propolis in the repair of sulcoplasties by the modified Kanzanjian technique: Cytological and clinical evalution." *Journal of the Nihon University School of Dentistry.* Vol. 36 (1994): 102–111.

Mahran, L.G. et al. "The protective effect of aqueous propolis extract on isolated rat hepatocytes against carbon tetrachloride toxicity." *Drugs Under Experimental and Clinical Research.* Vol. 22 (1996): 309–316.

Mirzoeva, O.K. and Calder, P.C. "The effect of propolis and its components on eicosanoid production during the inflammatory response." *Prostaglandins, Leukotrienes, and Essential Fatty Acids.* Vol. 55 (1996): 441–449.

Scheller, S. et al. "Ethanol extract of propolis (EEP) and dolomite potentiates the immunostimulatory effect of Biostymine and Levamisole in chronic bronchitis." *Pharmacology (Life Science Advances).* Vol. 14 (1995): 5–10.

——— "Ethanolic extract of propolis (EEP), a natural antioxidant, prolongs life span of male and female mice." *Pharmacology (Life Science Advances).* Vol. 13 (1994): 123–125.

Steinberg, D. et al. "Antibacterial effect of propolis and honey on oral bacteria." *American Journal of Dentistry.* Vol. 9 (1996): 236–239.

Honey

Ali, A.T.M. and Al-Swayeh. "Natural honey prevents ethanol-induced increased vascular permeability changes in the rat stomach." *Journal of Ethnopharmacology.* Vol. 55 (1997): 231–238.

Allen, K. et al. "A survey of the antibacterial activity of some New Zealand honeys." *Journal of Pharmacy and Pharmacology.* Vol. 43 (1991): 817–822.

al Somal, N.A. et al. "Susceptibility of Helicobacter pylori to the antibacterial activity of manuka honey." *Journal of the Royal Society of Medicine.* Vol. 87 (1994): 9–12.

Al-Waili, N.S. and Saloom, K.Y. "Effects of topical honey on post-operative wound infections due to gram positive and gram negative bacteria following Caesarean sections and hysterectomies." *European Journal of Medical Research.* Vol. 4 (1999): 126–130.

Cooper, R.A. et al. "Antibacterial activity of honey against strains of Staphylococcus aureus from infected wounds." *Journal of the Royal Society of Medicine.* Vol. 92 (1999): 283–285.

Frankel, S. et al. "Antioxidant capacity and correlated characteristics of 14 unifloral honeys." *Journal of Apicultural Research.* Vol. 37

(1998): 27–31.

Haffejee, I.E. and Moosa, A. "Honey in the treatment of infantile gastroenteritis." *British Medical Journal.* Vol. 290 (1985): 1866–1867.

——— "Why honey is effective as a medicine. Its use in modern medicine." *Bee World.* Vol. 80 (1999): 80–92.

Subrahmanyam, M. "Honey impregnated gauze versus polyurethane film (OpSite) in the treatment of burns—a prospective randomised study." *British Journal of Plastic Surgery.* Vol. 46 (1993): 322–323.

——— "Honey-impregnated gauze versus amniotic membrane in the treatment of burns." *Burns.* Vol. 20 (1994): 331–333.

Vardi, A. et al. "A local application of honey for treatment of neonatal postoperative wound infection." *Acta Paediatrica.* Vol. 87 (1998): 429–432.

Royal Jelly

Abd-Alla, M.S. et al. "Antimicrobial potency of royal jelly collected from queen cells at different larval stages." *Annals of Agricultural Science (Cairo).* Vol. 40 (1995): 597–608.

Al-Muffarej, S.I. and El-Sarag, M.S.A. "Effects of royal jelly on the humoral antibody response and blood chemistry of chickens." *Journal of Applied Animal Research.* Vol. 12 (1997): 41–47.

Fujiwara, S. et al. "A potent antibacterial protein in royal jelly." *Journal of Biological Chemistry.* Vol. 265 (1990): 11333–11337.

Iannuzzi, J. "Royal Jelly: Mystery Food, In three Parts." *American Bee Journal.* Vol. 8 (1990): 532–534, 587–589, 659–662.

Kim, J.G. and Son, J.H. "The quantity of superoxide dismutase (SOD) in fresh royal jelly." *Korean Journal of Apiculture.* Vol. 11 (1996): 8–12.

Lecker, G. et al. "Components of royal jelly II. The lipid fraction, hydrocarbons and sterols." *Journal of Apicultural Research.* Vol. 21 (1982): 178–184.

Shen, X. et al. "Effects of lyophilized royal jelly on experimental hyperlipidemia and thrombosis." *Chinese Journal of Preventive Medicine.* Vol. 29 (1995): 27–29.

Vittek, J. "Effect of royal jelly on serum lipids in experimental animals and humans with atherosclerosis." *Experientia.* Vol. 51 (1995): 927–935.

Yonekura, M. "Characterization and physiological function of royal jelly proteins." *Honeybee Science.* Vol. 19 (1998): 15–22.

[1] Bonvehi, J. S. and Jorda, R. E., 1997. Samples dried prior to analysis, losing over 10% water.

[2] Southern Testing and Research Labs Inc. certified chemical analysis, 1992 (provided by Bruce Brown, CC Pollen Co.).

[3] Covance Laboratories, Inc. certified chemical analysis, 2000 (provided by R. S. Gordon and M. Goldberg, Morrison School of Agribusiness and Management, Arizona State University East).

[4] Linskens, H. F. and Jorde, W., 1997.

sources

for bee products:
Natural Factors
3655 Bonneville Place
Burnaby, BC
V3N 4S9
1-800-663-8900

CC Pollen Co.
3627 E. Indian School Rd.
Suite 209
Phoenix, AZ 85018
Tel: 1-800-875-0096

Chris's Honey Yard
Holistic Allergy Control
Honey Pure &
Unpastuerized
Pollen Propolis Cappings
7108-152nd Street
Surrey, BC   V3S 3L8
Tel: (604) 599-7292
Fax: (604) 599-7265

**New Path Natural
Foods**
Distributed by Christmas
Natural Foods (Wholesalers)
Ltd.
#201-8173-128th Street
Surrey, BC V3W 4G1
Tel: (604) 591-8881
Fax: (604) 597-1784
www. christmasnatural-
foods.com

**Physiocorp Nutritional
Supplements**
4720-99 Street
Edmonton, Alberta
T6E 5H5
Tel: (780) 448-2220
Fax: (780) 448-0364
Toll Free: 1-800-465-3489

Comvita
91 Rylander Blvd
Scarborough, Ontario
M1B 5M5
Tel: (416) 808-4200
Fax: (416) 284-2725
Toll Free: 1-888-462-6852

Comvita
Old Couch Road
Bay of Plenty 3071
New Zealand
Tel: 64-7-5331426
Fax: 64-7-5331118
info@comvita.com

for natural oils
**Omega Nutrition of
Canada, Inc.**
1924 Franklin Street
Vancouver BC V5L 1R2
604–253–4677
800–661–3529

Omega–Life, Inc.
15355 Woodridge Road
Brookfield, WI 53005
(414) 786–2070
1–800–328–3529
(1–800–EAT–FLAX)

Barlean's
4936 Lake Terrell Road
Ferndale WA 982480
(306) 384-0485
1-800-445-3529

**Stoney Creek Oil
Products Pty. Ltd**
Talbot, Victoria,
Australia 3371
Tel: (03) 5463 2340

Thank you to "Chris's Honey Yard" for the use of his
facilities as a photoshoot location.

Remedies and supplements mentioned in this book are
available at quality health food stores and nutrition centers.

First published in 2000 by
alive **books**
7436 Fraser Park Drive
Burnaby BC V5J 5B9
(604) 435–1919
1-800–661–0303

Book Design:
   Liza Novecoski
Artwork:
   Terence Yeung
   Raymond Cheung
Food Styling/Recipe Development:
   Fred Edrissi
Photography:
   Edmond Fong
   (except when credited otherwise)
Photo Editing:
   Sabine Edrissi-Bredenbrock
Editing:
   Sandra Tonn

Canadian Cataloguing in
Publication Data

C. Leigh Broadhurst PhD
   Health and Healing
   with Bee Products

(*alive* Natural Health Guides, 28
ISSN 1490-6503)
ISBN 1-55312-031-0

Printed in Canada

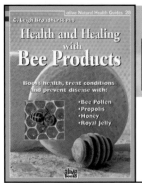

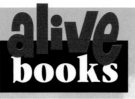

Natural
Your best source of

Self-Help Information

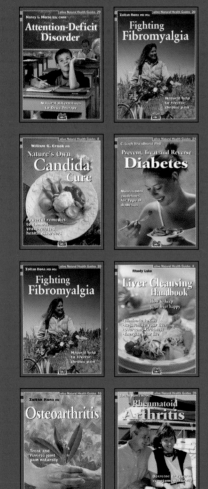

Healing Foods & Herbs

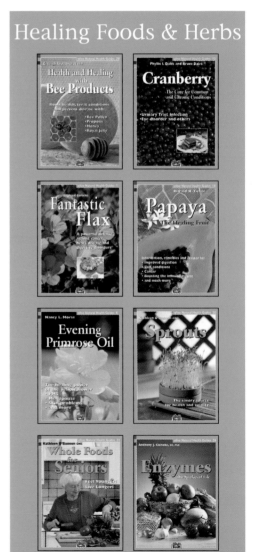

expert authors • easy-to-read information • tasty recipes